Freedom to Move

Movement and Dance for People with Intellectual Disabilities

Kim Dunphy

BA GradDip(Movement and Dance) MEd(Dance)

Jenny Scott

BA GradDip(Movement and Dance)

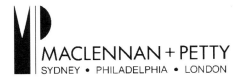

MACLENNAN + PETTY

SYDNEY • PHILADELPHIA • LONDON

First published 2003
MacLennan + Petty Pty Limited
Suite 405,152 Bunnerong Road
Eastgardens NSW 2036
www.maclennanpetty.com.au
© MacLennan + Petty Pty Limited

The National Library of Australia
Cataloguing-in-Publication data:

> Dunphy, Kim Frances.
> Freedom to move : movement and dance for people with
> intellectual disabilities.
>
> Bibliography.
> Includes index.
> ISBN 0 86433 185 1.
>
> 1. Dance therapy. 2. People with mental disabilities. I.
> Scott, Jenny, 1964- . II. Title.
>
> 616.8913

Printed and bound in Australia

Dedication

To the people who have inspired our journey through dance - especially my dance mothers, Phillipa Davern, Merilyn Byrne, Karen Bond and Hilary Crampton and my real mother Annette Dunphy

Kim Dunphy

My friends at BreakOut, The Oakleigh Centre for People with Intellectual Disabilities, St John of God–Brimbank Disability Support Services, Interact Learning Centre and Christopher Nolan. You have all shown me what it means to really dance.

Jenny Scott

Acknowledgments

Thank you for your valuable assistance and support to our families, John, Tessa and Lex Toumbourou (Kim), and Michael McGirr and Coralie Scott (Jenny), and to Debbie Lee, Dr Karen Bond, Christopher Brown, Lyn Dowling, Vicki Kirwin, Karina Doughty, Teri McNeil, Jean Kicks and Lawrence Turnbull from St David's Church, Moorabbin, Jutta Goodall, Andrea Weyman-Jones, Lisa George, parents and carers of BreakOut members.

Photos by Lyn Dowling with the exception of pages 28, 48, 63, *90, 110, 118, 119, 128, 131, 132, 139, 146, 147, 148, 161, *168, 181, 195.

* Photos by Sarah Lynch

Contents

Foreword

Freedom to Move has all the makings of a high quality professional development text. It is philosophical and practical, comprehensive and detailed, and is relevant to a broad readership within the fields of disability and dance-based performing arts. The authors begin by locating their backgrounds as dancers, teachers, and socially conscious human beings in a shared worldview that affirms the right of people with disabilities to enjoy the fulfilment and 'freedom' available through artistic expression. Then, over ten generous chapters, the writers present content and methods for a developmentally sound approach to dance advocacy, program planning, group facilitation, and evaluation. The authors' model of evaluation is innovative in its emphasis on reflective practice and attention to the multiple perspectives of all who may become involved in the dynamic realm of 'dance for the (so called) disabled,' including participants, families/carers, organisations, funding bodies, and program staff. Overall *Freedom to Move* inspires confidence. It is based on the extensive professional knowledge of two committed practitioners, including their currency with relevant theory and research. The text is enlivened with stories and photographs from the 'lived experience' of the authors and their clients.

Freedom to Move honours human diversity and its expression through dance. Welcome to the 21st century!

Karen E. Bond, Ph.D.
Temple University
Philadelphia, Pennsylvania

About the authors

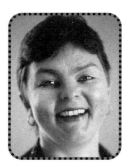

Kim Dunphy *BA GradDip(Movement and Dance) MEd(Dance)* is a community dance educator who has worked extensively in the field of disability. Kim currently lectures in dance and education at various tertiary institutions including Box Hill Institute and Melbourne University. Her experience includes leading groups for adults and children in hospitals, training and community centres and in mainstream and special schools in Melbourne, country Victoria and the USA. Kim is past director of the community-based BreakOut Dance Group, and a committee member of the Dance Therapy Association of Australia.

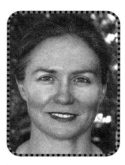

Jenny Scott *BA GradDip(Movement and Dance)* is a dance teacher and therapist who leads dance groups for people with disabilities in day training centres, community centres and hospitals in Melbourne. She is the current director of BreakOut Dance Group. Jenny has run many training programs and professional development activities for disability and education staff throughout Australia. She also performs as part of the integrated movement theatre group Weave.

Preface

Freedom to Move is a how-to book for leaders of dance/movement groups for people with intellectual disabilities. The book includes:

- discussion of the value of dance for people with disabilities, descriptions of other successful programs and a summary of relevant research

- information on health and fitness issues for people with intellectual disabilities

- practical aspects of running a session, including ideas for warm-up, themes, improvisation, choreography and performance using a Laban-based creative approach

- lesson plans for groups with different needs, including children, children in mainstream settings, people with high support needs and older adults

- strategies for running groups for people with intellectual disabilities

- strategies for planning and evaluating programs

- a list of relevant organisations

- discography of ideas for music to use in sessions

- a bibliography detailing relevant references in community arts and arts therapies, dance and dance therapy, disability and fitness.

The book can be used as a foundation for newcomers to the field, or as a professional development resource for those with more experience. Most of the ideas, techniques and strategies can be used with different age groups –children, adults or seniors – and in a range of settings, including classrooms, dance studios, gymnasiums and day centres. They are useful for small and large groups, and require little formal dance training on the part of the group leader. They do, however, require a group leader who has a love of movement and dance, group management/teaching skills and a desire to make a positive contribution to the lives of individuals with intellectual disabilities.

We have written *Freedom to Move* as an introduction for people wanting to work in the very rewarding area of dance and movement for people with intellectual disabilities. Both of us have worked extensively in this field, in a range of settings including special schools, community centres, day-training centres and hospitals. For some years, we have also directed BreakOut, a community-based group that specialises in creative dance classes for people with intellectual disabilities, based in the south-eastern suburbs of Melbourne, Australia.

We have often been asked by dance teachers, students and therapists for advice and resources on working in this field. We decided to document our work as a way of sharing our experiences and assisting others to find a place where they can start. This seemed particularly important as there are currently few resources on the specific topic of movement and dance for people with intellectual disabilities. Our bibliography lists a few relevant titles including Gina Levete's *No Handicap to Dance* (extremely useful for ideas for movement/drama improvisation activities), Guthrie and Roydhouse's *Come and Join The Dance* (an excellent program for working with special needs children), Adam Benjamin's *Making An Entrance* (more specifically focused on physical disability issues and performance) and *Positive/Negative* (readings on integrated dance).

We have always been passionate about dance and its value as a means of self-expression, and as a way of exploring our individuality. As adults, we chose dance as a career because it combined our need for passion, joy and creativity with work that made a contribution to the lives of others. In some ways the decision to work with people with disabilities was an easy one because they often have limited life opportunities and are therefore often the most appreciative of new experiences.

Our extensive training in different dance styles - including classical ballet, modern dance, folk dance, spiritual dance, creative dance, improvisation and performing, has informed and enriched our work with disabled students, and provided a range of choices and artistic elements to draw from. We have also both had training in dance therapy and draw on dance therapy principles and research to inform our work.

It is possible, however, for professionals from different backgrounds to work successfully in this field with much less dance training. One of the aims of this book is to provide ideas and stimuli for those who work in the field of disability but who may not have a particularly strong dance background. When we run in-service training for teachers or care workers without dance backgrounds we dance as little as possible ourselves in order to demonstrate that finely-honed technical skills are not necessary to provide an enjoyable and creative experience for a class or group.

We have also written this book for dance specialists or therapists who may be inexperienced in the field of intellectual disability, but who need ideas on how to apply their artform to a new clientele.

One particularly strong influence for us has been the Laban-based dance education and therapy training that we both undertook at the University of Melbourne. These graduate courses, led by Dr Karen Bond, were significant as they provided training for people to work outside the traditional performance-based dance milieu. They also paved the way for the proliferation of dance therapy activity throughout Australia.

Laban-based movement accommodates bodies and minds of varying capacities. Unlike a technique-based dance style in which a student must perform preordained movements, a creative dance class does not require a student to have particular movement, sensory or communication skills. The challenge for the teacher or group leader in a Laban-based class is to extend the participant to and beyond their current capability and to assist them to be the most expressive that they have the desire to be.

Why work with people with intellectual disabilities?

There are many reasons why we are drawn to use dance as an expressive medium with people with intellectual disabilities. One of the main incentives is the sheer pleasure of working with people who can be so immediate and open in their responses. If a group leader/teacher presents an activity that is not sufficiently engaging to a class of people with intellectual disabilities, they won't quietly co-operate for the session and then decide not to come back the following week. They will demand that the activity be modified on the spot! Conversely, if the group leader gets it right, the group is likely to participate with great gusto.

We are continually delighted by the creative acts and moments of sheer artistry in our work with people with intellectual disabilities. We often wish we had the video camera recording those moments for posterity. Of course, there are other days when that spark is missing, when class members or staff are out of sorts, and it is just plain ordinary, but overall there are many magical moments. This is perhaps because people with intellectual disabilities often have less awareness and therefore fewer concerns regarding the perceptions of others. This can be the reverse experience of working with teenagers, for example, whose intense self-consciousness and concern about self-image can really inhibit creativity and spontaneity.

The best work a person can do is that which utilises one's own talents while also making a contribution to the lives of others. For most of us, it is also important to be trained for work that can contribute to our livelihood, or it will be a short-lived career. While the fields of dance therapy and community dance continue to grow, it remains an ongoing challenge to find paid work that makes use of one's skills, training and experience. However, services for people with disabilities are expanding, especially those that are community-based and aim to increase leisure and expressive opportunities. Paid work in this area has presented itself to us on a fairly regular basis. For both of us, it was most difficult in the beginning before we were experienced or had become known in the field. The strategy of offering our services as volunteer workers during placements as part of our dance education studies led to paid work that expanded into more opportunities.

We have led sessions in agencies including psychogeriatric hospitals, community centres, day training centres and special schools. We have also created our own opportunities by expanding our own group and approaching agencies ourselves. For Kim, the first opportunity for paid work leading a dance program for disabled clients came when she was employed as a residential support worker. Jenny was able to secure funding for a dance program with a client she first worked for when she was a graduate dance student volunteer. More information about the way various programs have been set up can be found in Chapter 8.

We hope that as a result of writing this book there will be more leaders successfully running dance programs for people with disabilities, and contributing to their health and wellbeing, fitness and community connectedness. Good luck!

Kim Dunphy
Jenny Scott
Melbourne
October 2002

Chapter 1

The value of dance for people with intellectual disabilities

Why dance?

Over the past few decades there have been significant changes in society's attitudes to and treatment of people with intellectual disabilities. While it was once widely regarded that those with intellectual disabilities should live in segregated institutions, it is now generally accepted that participation in mainstream community life is more appropriate and humane. This social and political change has resulted in a greater range of possibilities for people with disabilities in their home, work, social and cultural lives.

One area that has developed along with the overall expansion of life opportunities for people with disabilities is that of artistic participation and expression. There has been an increase in the number and variety of opportunities in the performing arts for people with disabilities, including dance, over the past twenty years. Researchers and practitioners have documented their practice and outcomes for participants in various dance/movement-based programs, including psycho-therapeutic dance therapy, creative movement, improvisation and disability arts as performance.

This chapter provides a summary and comparison of these approaches and an assessment of their suitability for people with intellectual disabilities.

Community involvement: Changes in attitude to people with intellectual disabilities

Current health and community service policies for people with disabilities emphasise concepts of a good life, self-determination and involvement in everyday family and community life. This view has gradually developed over the past 30 years or so, in line with other social changes that promote equality of opportunity for all people. The principles of an 'ordinary life' were set out by the King's Fund in the United Kingdom in 1980 (Carnaby 1999) as part of the concept of 'normalisation'. The concept of normalisation for people with learning disabilities include these principles:

- the right to the same opportunities in the community as others
- greater independence as part of an age appropriate lifestyle
- involvement in decisions affecting their own lives
- provision of services that are local, accessible and comprehensive.

This philosophical view has its historical roots in the normalisation, independent living and disability rights movement of the 1960s and 1970s (Nirje, 1969; Wolfensberger, 1972) and the self-advocacy/self-help movement of the 1980s (Driedger, 1989). The current State Disability Plan, a new Victorian government policy for people with disabilities, entitled *The Key to Inclusion*, has a similar theme. This document describes the new era where people with a disability participate and have the same rights, opportunities and responsibilities as all citizens. The vision is for a stronger and more inclusive community where diversity is embraced and celebrated and where everyone has the same opportunities to participate in the life of the community (Department of Human Services, 2002).

These views are radically different from earlier practices relating to people with disabilities. Fifty years ago, people who gave birth to disabled children were encouraged to place them in institutions and forget about them. Huge establishments such as Kew Cottages and St Nicholas in Melbourne, Australia, were long-term homes to people with disabilities. They led institutionalised lives, disconnected from their families and the mainstream community.

Journalist Rosemary West described a poignant first meeting with a sister she had never met before, when they were both in their late middle age (West, 1996). Verna, who has Down syndrome, was placed in Kew Cottages as a young child by her 18-year-old unmarried mother, and grew up never knowing members of her extended family who lived less than an hour's drive away. When Rosemary learned of her sister's existence, courtesy of a dedicated staff member of that institution, she sought her out and the women were able to develop a sisterly relationship for the first time. The 1988 movie *Rainman*, starring Dustin Hoffman, depicted a similar practice that took place in the United States. In the movie, a young man rediscovers his autistic brother, Raymond, after his father's death. Raymond had been placed in an institution following the untimely death of the brothers' young mother.

These significant changes in social policy have meant that the lives of people with intellectual disabilities are now much improved. Families in many western countries are now given support to bring up children with disabilities at home, and involve them in community life as much as possible. Agencies such as the pioneering Noah's Ark Resource Centre, Fostercare and Interchange programs, offer families a range of services to assist with the extra demands of children with special needs. The consequences of these changes are very significant. The health of people with disabilities has markedly improved, as exemplified by the huge change in life expectancy for people with Down syndrome that has occurred over the past 30 years. In the early 1900s, the average life expectancy was only nine years. By the 1950s, most people with Down syndrome were reaching their 50s and today one in ten may expect to live to 70 years of age (Selikowitch, 1992). The contributing factors to this change include medical intervention, the move towards a more normal lifestyle within the community rather than institutionalisation, and the availability of a range of behavioural and social interventions (Brown, 1995). Medical researchers Yang, Rasmussen and Friedman (2002), also attribute this dramatic improvement, in part, to the practice of de-institutionalisation, because children growing up at home benefit from better healthcare, nutrition and lifestyles. Numerous studies indicate the positive impact of a stimulating home environment on the development of young people with Down syndrome, including regular participation in such activities as family outings, club memberships, vacations and other age-appropriate activities (Shepperdson 1995; Berry, Groeneweg, Gibson, Brown, 1984).

For adults, living options have changed a lot too. Large institutions have gradually been closed down and replaced with smaller home-style residences in which disabled adults ideally have opportunities for more self-directed lives. Disability specialists work with clients to find employment, leisure and social options that match individuals' interests, abilities and life stage. Wehmeyer and Schwartz describe the 'growing mindfulness in the fields of disability services, rehabilitation, education and psychology of the need to promote self-determination for individuals with intellectual disabilities' (1998, p. 3). Brown (1995) found that many adults with developmental disabilities achieved a 'startling' increase in self-image when they had opportunities to select activities they wished to become involved in. He believes that 'a stimulating environment with broad-ranging activities in leisure … is essential', and its impacts are likely to be 'improved health, expanded motivation and improved self-image for individuals' (1995, p. 46).

Agencies all over Australia are working to increase community and leisure opportunities for people with disabilities. In Victoria, the state government's Access for All Abilities project collaborates with mainstream sport and leisure providers to enhance opportunities for people with disabilities. VicsRapid promotes participation and achievement through sport and recreation, while Arts Access and its sister organisations in each state play a major role in developing artistic opportunities for people who are disadvantaged. This development has a parallel in many other countries, as exemplified by Benjamin's (2001) astonishingly long list of groups who practise arts that are inclusive of people with all kinds of disabilities.

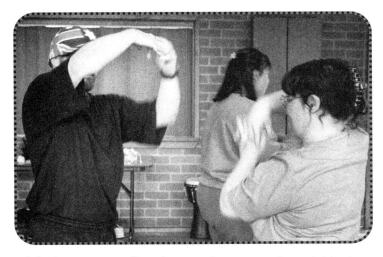

The concept of the importance of involvement in community activities is not only applicable to people with intellectual disabilities. Theorists from many different fields including health, sociology, arts and culture describe similar concepts with regard to the quality of life and wellbeing of all people. Research by sociologists Catalano and Hawkins (1996) indicates that one of most significant factors in a psychologically healthy life is the need for a sense of community and belonging, which can be achieved by enjoyable shared activity and positive experiences with peers, friends and family. According to sociologist Richard Eckersley, psychological wellbeing is closely related to meaning in life, which is cultivated by 'membership in groups, dedication to a cause and clear life goals', among other things (1999, p. 18).

Indicators of social capital, as measured by community health researchers Bullen and Onyx (1998), include participation in local community, pro-activity in a social context, neighbourhood connections, and connections with family and friends. These recommendations point to the value of participation in a community-based recreational activity such as a dance program, which includes opportunities for group membership, enjoyable shared activity and participation in a community activity.

Rita enjoys participation in a group at BreakOut

Rita is an older adult with autism and a moderate intellectual disability whose language is confined mostly to mentions of her favourite foods and some limited echolalia (automatic repetition of words and phrases). Rita's care workers believe that participation in a dance program like BreakOut is important for her because it is one of the few activities she enjoys that includes physical exercise and a connection with others through eye and body contact. Otherwise, Rita's preferred pastime is purchasing and eating her favourite foods.

BreakOut class is also a time when Rita can really indulge her passion and remarkable talent for singing. Her capacity for echolalia functions really well with song words. Rita can listen to a song, and, if it takes her fancy, repeat it with perfect pitch. She also has an enormous repertoire of songs that she can sing flawlessly, karaoke style, whenever she really enjoys music that is being played. Rita's favourites are always on hand at BreakOut, to add motivation for the days when it is difficult to get her to cooperate with others and focus fully on class activities. The right music acts as a kind of trigger for participation, ensuring that Rita is at least involved enough to sing along. On good days, when Rita is enthused enough to join the group in dance activities, her eyes shine, her face beams and she sings along excitedly to the music accompanying the session.

Value of arts participation: Health and wellbeing

There is evidence that participation in arts is a factor in the development and sustainment of health and wellbeing. Cultural theorist Jon Hawkes (2001) argues for the value of arts participation at a community level:

> [A]ctive community participation in arts practice is an essential component of a healthy and sustainable society … arts practice not only opens up fantastic vistas of community expressivity but also … profoundly contributes to the development of community.

Williams (2001) describes studies in Australia and the United Kingdom that show social and educational outcomes of involvement in community arts programs, including:

◎ development of community networks and generation of greater social cohesion
◎ generation of a sense of community pride
◎ generation of greater tolerance of different cultures and lifestyles
◎ prevention of crime or a decrease in antisocial behaviour

- ◉ improved sense of community confidence and wellbeing
- ◉ pursuit of further education or networks leading to employment
- ◉ improved consultation leading to better design or planning of public facilities.

She also comments that:

> there is a large body of evidence that the major residual benefits from community-based arts programs come from developing social and human capital, that is, in how these experiences can develop new insights, connections, skills and knowledge which influence changes to people's attitudes and behaviour (2001, p.2).

In the landmark US study, *Champions of Change: The Impact of the Arts on Learning*, Fiske (1999) finds that the arts provide young people with authentic learning experiences that engage their minds, hearts and bodies. The study documents how involvement in quality arts learning experiences engages young people in ways that other experiences do not, in that they:

- ◉ reach young people who are not otherwise being reached
- ◉ reach young people in ways that they are not otherwise being reached
- ◉ connect young people to themselves and each other
- ◉ provide learning opportunities for the adults in the lives of young people
- ◉ connect learning experiences to the world of real work.

Fiske (1999) discovered that out of school arts programs for disadvantaged youth were more beneficial in terms of learning and achievement for young people than programs in sport or community involvement. Corkum et al. (2001), writing from an Australian perspective, outline the benefits of participation in the arts that include a greater sense of wellbeing, more community connectedness, less depression and better physical health.

In the case of people with intellectual disabilities, a limited range of studies indicate the benefits of arts participation. For example, therapist /researchers Zagelbaum and Rubino (1991) reported on the social and interactional benefits of participation in a therapeutic arts program for a client with serious behavioural challenges, as well as psychiatric and profound intellectual disabilities. Over a ten-month period of participation in the multi-art (dance/movement, music and art) program, the woman showed significant improvements in social functioning, including social communication, social skills, reduced hostility, eye contact, group participation and communication.

Dance has the additional dimension of providing opportunities for artistic expression through movement. DanceAbility, a form of contact improvisation that facilitates exploration of movement possibilities even for those with severely restricted mobility and communication, offers participants a unique experience. A DanceAbility workshop attendee described the significance of this experience for her. This young woman, who was normally strapped in a wheelchair because of her very limited movement, felt that the annual DanceAbility weekend in her town was 'the best day of her year', providing her with 'freedom and acceptance' that was not part of her everyday life (Dunphy, 1999a).

The following story indicates a transformation in participant Charlie that occurred during participation in a dance/drama program.

Charlie, the Tin Man: Transformation through dramatic expression

Charlie was a tall, solidly built man in his late twenties who had a moderate intellectual disability and very limited verbal communication. Throughout most of the Act It Out dance/drama sessions, Charlie was a fairly inert participant, largely because of difficulties he was experiencing with his medication. He found it difficult to stay awake, even in morning classes, and very often snoozed off when he got a chance to sit down. Act It Out sessions would always begin with vigorous physical activities to stimulate energy in an attempt to help keep Charlie involved and active.

When the parts for the end-of-year show (excerpts from *The Wizard of Oz*) were being cast, Charlie seemed the perfect choice for the part of the Tin Man, as there was little need for dialogue and his tall, rigid physique matched the physical requirements of the part perfectly. Charlie appeared to enjoy his 'script', which required him to utter a loud squeak each time the oil can was applied to his body. He smiled broadly whenever he managed to squeak loudly enough for the audience to hear. The highlight of Charlie's role was his transformation from the rusted-stiff suit of armour to the free-flowing friend who accompanied Dorothy along the Yellow Brick Road.

Charlie worked hard to change his movements from his usual heavy-weight stillness as the pre-oiled Tin Man to a freer travelling movement after the oiling. He achieved this through gradual movement isolations of body parts; arms, shoulders, legs, feet, head and neck, before re-integrating all of these movements and gradually propelling himself into forward gear for the journey to Oz. Fortunately, Charlie had a supportive co-star in Dorothy, who was able to co-actively assist those body parts that stuck a little!

Creative expression: The creative potential of people with intellectual disabilities

A view commonly held by experts in the early and mid-twentieth century was that people with intellectual disabilities were inherently uncreative because they were limited to concrete thought processes, and therefore not capable of abstract or symbolic thinking (for example, Kounin 1941a, 1941b, 1948; Lewin 1935). Stamatelos and Mott (1985) describe a notion espoused by such writers, that creativity is related systematically to intelligence, so that one assumes people with low IQs would be equally low in creativity. Until quite recently, people with intellectual disabilities experienced very limited lifestyles and opportunities as a result of such beliefs.

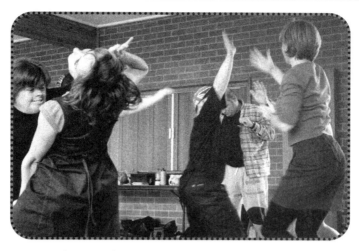

Those ideas have since been refuted by numerous researchers and clinicians including Lowenfeld and Brittian, 1964; Stabler, Stabler and Karger, 1977; Stamatelos and Mott, 1983a; with Stamatelos and Mott describing them as 'pervasive myths' (1985, p. 101). More recent research has indicated the creative potential of people with intellectual disabilities. Stamatelos and Mott (1985) contended that both abstract thought and the use of symbolic processes occur in persons with developmental delays, thus indicating a capacity for creative acts. They devised a program to facilitate the creativity of people with intellectual disabilities based on humanistic theoretical framework. Habilitative Arts Therapy provides opportunities for people with intellectual disabilities to demonstrate creative thinking through the creative arts modalities of music, movement, visual art and writing (Stamatelos and Mott, 1983a).

In our experience, the creative potential of people with intellectual disabilities is evident. The following story describes BreakOut member Jon's unique choreography.

Jon, the Eagle Man, enjoys creative expression through dance

One of our BreakOut students often demonstrates his identification with nature and the world of birds in his eagle dance. Jon and his family are nature lovers who live close by the beach. They often walk down there in the early morning to observe the local bird life. Jon's original choreography, which has become a theme of his creative life, represents himself as his favourite bird, the eagle, based on his observation of eagles and other birds of prey. Motifs from this dance often appear in Jon's improvisations – a strong upright stance, body balanced on the balls of the feet, arms opened wide, poses held still like the eagle as it glides on the breeze searching for food.

While the capacity for creative expression is not necessarily lacking in people with intellectual disabilities, opportunities to experiment and explore ideas often are. This is particularly so for people who have spent much of their lives in an institution. We have become aware of a distinction in expressive potential between generations of people with disabilities; older adults who have lived much of their lives out of sight and separate from family and community life are much less able to experiment and explore ideas than younger people who have been encouraged to take a place in the community. This difference parallels significant health improvements resulting from life outside institutions, as discussed earlier. The story of Jessie and Tabetha below exemplifies a contrast in creative and expressive capability between members of these two generations.

Jessie and Tabetha: The value of community participation and possibilities beyond disability

Jessie has attended weekly classes for older adults at BreakOut for almost five years. She is now in her sixties and is part of a generation of people with disabilities who have spent most of their lives in institutions without any access to early intervention or community programs. Jessie has Down syndrome and her speech and social interactive skills are limited, though she has great strength of character and enjoys taking the lead so she can direct the dance session her way. Jessie's focus is often centred on putting away chairs and packing up all the props. Her favourite saying is, 'We need to put it away now'.

For some time we thought that Jessie's persistence in putting away chairs and props during sessions was something she did to assert her individual power in the situation. During one session we had occasion to rethink this view and suddenly had an insight into her behaviour. This particular day Jessie was the only group member to turn up for the session, which meant that for the whole hour the group comprised Jessie, myself (Jenny, as group leader) and our assistant, Karina.

Jessie began by putting away the chairs we had carefully placed in a circle to begin the session. She then told us we needed to put away the scarves we had also carefully placed in the centre of the circle and insisted on packing them up into a storage bag. We decided that the only alternative to packing up and going home ourselves was to respond playfully to Jessie's 'packing up' regime. We followed Jessie's lead by unpacking all the props so that she had lots of things to put away. This included a very long skein of wool. The three of us played for about 20 minutes with the wool, finding different shapes to make as we slowly wound it up into a nice neat ball to be put away.

On reflection, and by paying more attention to Jessie's frequently repeated words, 'Put it away now', we realised that Jessie had difficulty with the concept of playful interaction with objects. As we brought other items such as a bag and chair into the improvisation, Jessie seemed only to be able to relate to them according to their everyday function. She became frustrated when we pretended that the bag was a hat and demanded that it be used only to pack everything away.

We wondered whether this difficulty may have been related to a lack of opportunities for creative exploration through play, growing up with an intellectual disability in the 40s and 50s. We thought it likely that she had not had the opportunity to re-experience play through the role of parenting or as a care-giver to a child. It is possible that Jessie's life experience has limited her capacity to engage in play, and therefore restricted her imagination and spontaneity.

continued

In contrast, Tabetha is a woman in her early twenties who has benefited from her community's more enlightened approach to people with disabilities. As a consequence, she has been able to move beyond the restrictions that her disability could create. Tabetha's involvement in BreakOut is a good example of such a process. When Tabetha first started at BreakOut, her movement repertoire consisted of star jumps and stretches. Her aerobic style movement was two-dimensional and functional, with minimal flow quality and restricted expressive potential. Over the years that Tabetha has attended weekly classes and participated in performances her movement style has gradually expanded to include three-dimensional movement. There is noticeably more flow and experimentation in her use of body. Along with star jumps, Tabetha now includes spirals, curves and circles in her chosen movements. Sometimes she is so creatively inspired that she can work at different levels, choosing rolling and sliding along the floor as her contribution to warm-up improvisations.

Tabetha has also been encouraged to describe her movement. For example, when she was asked, 'What were you thinking of?' and 'What did you feel?' after one improvisation, Tabetha responded that she felt like a bird and that flying made her feel happy. Then quite spontaneously she told the group they were her friends and that she loved coming to BreakOut. Through discovering new movement, Tabetha was also able to explore her thoughts and feelings and had the opportunity to express them. Unlike many people of the older generation, Tabetha is finding possibilities beyond her disability.

Physical health and wellbeing: The contribution of participation in dance

In addition to the mental health and wellbeing benefits of involvement in arts activities, participation in dance programs also offers the physical benefits of weight-bearing exercise. While the same recommendation of 30 minutes a day of moderate exercise applies to people with intellectual disabilities as to others in the community (Beange, Lennox and Parmenter, 1999), exercise levels are generally low in this section of the population (Beange, McElduff and Baker, 1995). This is particularly concerning because exercise can have a positive impact on conditions that occur at a higher rate among people with intellectual disabilities than for the general population, such as cardiovascular disease (Beange, McElduff and Baker, 1995), obesity (Rimmer, 1993; Beange, McElduff and Baker, 1995; and Roizen, Luke, Sutton and Schoeller, 1995), chronic constipation (Cathels, 1993), osteoporosis (Center, Beange and McElduff, 1998) and respiratory disease (O'Brien et al., 1991). Depression is also a major concern, with Rowitz and Jurkowski (1995) reporting that the incidence of depression among people with intellectual disabilities was highest for those who reported doing no leisure activities (75 per cent) and lowest for people with greater than seven reported activities (9.59 per cent). They recommended development of recreational activities that include exercise.

Overall, the health of people with intellectual disabilities is far worse than the health of the general population. For example, they have higher mortality rates (1.7 up to 4.1 times the general population, depending on severity of disabilities according to Forssman and Akesson, 1970), especially those with Down syndrome, whose life expectancy is only 55 years (Strauss and Eyman, 1996).

Hayden (1998) suggests that opportunities for active and passive movement be provided for those with mobility limitations, given that immobility contributes to reduced life expectancy. Beange, Lennox and Parmenter (1999) recommend that 'the provision of exercise programs at a local level is a cost-effective way of improving health, and while many people with disabilities can participate in activities available for the general public, others will need special services' (p. 292). Beange, McElduff and Baker (1995) discuss lack of opportunity as one factor of a lack of exercise.

For people with disabilities, accessing appropriate exercise activities can be difficult. There are fewer options available and all kinds of obstacles. It is often difficult to know what a person might like when they have never had the chance to try it, when they can't speak, or when what they might like to do is not available at a level they can manage, or anywhere near where they live. Then there are the challenges with access (for example, getting in the door or into the toilet), challenges with attitude (for example, they might find something that interests them, but discover that the people there are not open to their participation), as well as the challenges of actually doing it.

Physical exercise that is intrinsically enjoyable is particularly important for people who may not have the cognitive capacity to understand the importance of exercise. Many of the mainstream population exercise not because they enjoy it or really want to do it, but because they are conscious of the negative consequences if they don't. For people without this awareness it is important to provide activities that are intrinsically enjoyable. A dance class has the benefits of being creative and social and many people find this enjoyable. Client participation is therefore more likely to be ongoing, with likelihood of better health outcomes.

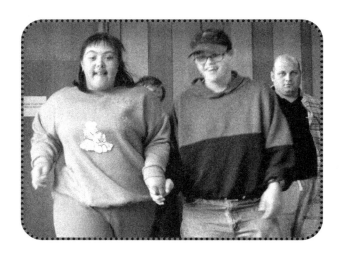

The health outcomes that can be gained from participation in dance programs have been compared favourably against more traditional fitness programs. Lasseter et al. (1989) found that a 12-year-old girl with cerebral palsy, mild intellectual disability and emotional problems experienced a more positive sense of self and a marked improvement in motor development after a 12-week dance treatment program. Bachman and Sluyter (1988) reported the positive effects of a program of aerobic dance for adult attendees at a day activity centre for intellectually disabled adults. Students engaging in exercise dance classes three times per week showed a decrease in inappropriate behaviours, including inappropriate vocalisations, repetitive movements and time off-task. Tipple (1975) documented improvements in posture, walking, general level of confidence and poise for female residents in an Ontario institution following a varied dance program that included ballet, tap, ballroom and acrobatic dance.

Therapy versus art: What is appropriate?

There has been considerable discussion about the relationship of dance therapy to other dance modalities in the field of intellectual disability. There is evidence of the value of dance therapy and of dance programs that have recreational, educational or performance focuses. Our experiences with people who have varying degrees of disability have led us to the view that all of these can be suitable modalities, with the appropriate choice being dependent on four factors: the clients' support needs, the clients' ability and interest in dance, the contract between group leader and client/s and the skills of the group leader.

A number of studies document the benefits of dance therapy with children and adults. Loman and Merman (1996) described the positive outcomes of a dance therapy process for a four-year-old boy with autism. The process of attunement initiated by the therapist resulted in improved communication, increased trust, more control over the environment and greater creativity in her young client.

Ohwaki (1976) described the positive impact of a dance therapy program on the body image of adult participants. Silk's (1989) dance movement therapy program offered opportunities for participants to make choices, develop ideas and strengthen leadership capacities through dance experiences. The clients in Silk's program gained skills in a variety of areas as well as improving their fitness. Loman and Merman (1996) proposed the view that developmental dance/dance therapy is the most suitable dance modality for patients with poor cognitive skills and language ability. As evidence, they described a successful dance therapy session that provided a group of developmentally delayed and emotionally disturbed adults with opportunities for self-expression, and noted the development of improved impulse control, coping and social skills.

Is it therapy or creative dance?

Creative dance has been described as 'a free approach to the art of body movement which gives everyone opportunity to discover for himself his own forms of movement expression according to his physiological and psychological needs', (Mettler, 1990, p. 95). This style of dance seems to be a popular option for groups with intellectual disabilities, as documented by practitioners such as Lishman (1985), Silk (1989), Guthrie and Roydhouse (1988), Boswell (1993) and Schlusser (2000). It is also the approach we use with our groups.

There does, however, seem to be considerable overlap between the various writers' concepts of dance therapy and creative dance. Guthrie and Roydhouse (1988), for example, describe their dance program for children with special needs as a Laban-based 'creative approach to movement'. While the program offered creative movement experiences, the leader's aims seemed to be more therapeutic than artistic, in providing children with 'a wide range of sensory motor activities to stimulate growth and learning appropriate to meet the needs of each individual, whatever their stage of development or handicap' (p. 28). In the article referred to earlier, Silk reveals a similar dilemma, evidenced by her description of herself as a dance therapist and her program as dance therapy, while her article is entitled 'Creative movement for people who are developmentally delayed'.

Studies documenting outcomes of Laban-based creative dance programs seem to measure therapeutic outcomes. Laban pioneered the concept of 'free dance', allowing the dancer to move freely, without restrictions. (The Laban technique is explained in detail in Chapter 2.) Lishman (1985), for example, describes the 'many pervasive reasons' why a Laban-based creative movement program advanced the learning of children with developmental disabilities further than more structured programs like Doman-Delacato and perceptual-motor programs. These include freedom of individual inventiveness and creative expression, wider movement vocabulary, and an increased interest in and curiosity for learning. Boswell (1993) found that participation in a creative dance program improved the balance skills of children with mild intellectual disabilities more than a traditional gross motor program.

Many writers have addressed the distinction between the two modalities. Leventhal, in her 1980 article about children with special needs, describes the similarities, which include the fact that dance therapy and creative dance share basic tools: the moving body coping with force, time, space and flow. However, Leventhal believes that while dance therapy encourages self-expression as a process to attain emotional insight and interpretation and movement dialogue between the therapist and child, creative dance emphasises the building of technique and development of form. Her view is that dance therapy is the treatment of choice for children with learning disabilities.

Creative dance teacher Barbara Mettler recognises clear differences between creative dance and dance therapy. She believes that art and therapy have:

> entirely different goals and motivations …While the goal of therapy is the healing of illness, the goal of art is the creation of a satisfying form. Therapy is utilitarian, serving a purpose beyond itself … art serves no purpose other than providing joy in the creative work itself (1990, p. 96).

However, Mettler does comment that 'all art is, by its very nature, therapeutic … But therapy is a by-product of art, not its essential nature' (1990, p. 98).

In discussing the appropriateness of dance therapy for people with intellectual disabilities it must be considered that intellectual disability is not a condition that can be treated or healed through therapy, unlike psychological disorders that have traditionally been the domain of dance therapists. An intellectual disability is one characteristic of a person, one of the many that contribute to the make-up of an individual, but it is not one that necessarily needs curing or indeed can be cured. Some people with intellectual disabilities also have behavioural or

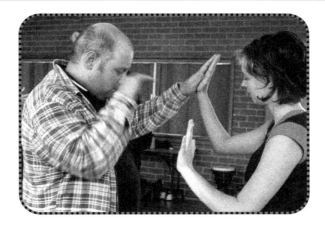

psychological conditions that can be assisted by therapy, but there are many others who simply have a lower than normal IQ. Thus, the role of a dance specialist working in this field could be to provide dance opportunities that contribute to participants' health and wellbeing in the same way that any recreational, educational or community-based dance program might.

Mainstream versus specialised options

Current philosophy in the field of disability services emphasises the importance of increased opportunities and an environment that is as unrestricted as possible. Opportunities for participation in dance are appropriate in this paradigm, affording people with disabilities access to recreation choices that any other person in the community might have. These may be mainstream or specialised, depending on the skill and functioning level of the participant. Many people with moderate to severe intellectual disabilities need more support than a mainstream option is likely to provide. Our own BreakOut Dance Group recognises and caters for the different needs of some individuals with disabilities and/or challenging behaviours. These include simplified communication, less emphasis on outcome, the provision of manageable challenges within a supportive environment and some physical care. However, many other people with intellectual disabilities are talented and creative performers who may be better served by more professional training and performing experiences.

Community arts approach

Participation in the arts for people with intellectual disabilities has the potential to be more than just a recreational activity, providing, in addition, an outlet for creative and expressive talents. Community art is a model of art-making that 'celebrates the diversity and talents of people in the community ... whose value is to build and express diverse community cultures, as part of the culture of wider society'. (Williams, 2001).

Numerous writers have described this kind of activity with their groups. Schlusser, for example, documented the deeply creative and artistic practices of the intellectually disabled members of her Stretch Theatre Company (2000). Lovis' experience with performers with intellectual disabilities in the Prime Movers Company led her to the observation that individual disabilities can 'inspire movement and speech inventions' of 'remarkable originality' (Lovis 1992, p. 34). Hugill encountered 'passion, commitment, brilliant capacities for clowning and intuitive comprehension of character subtleties', among intellectually disabled members of his company Theatre Unlimited (Hugill 1992).

Disability arts as professional performance

There is yet a further possibility, that participation in dance might develop beyond an enjoyable expression and performance at a community level into the creation of art of a professional standard. Over the last few decades there has been a considerable increase in the number of professional performing companies comprised of members with intellectual disabilities, or integrated groups of people with and without disabilities, all around the world. Anne Riordan (1989) described the evolution of the Sunrise Company performing group from a recreation program for intellectually disabled adults at the Work Activity Centre in Salt Lake City, Utah, USA. After an initial introduction to creative dance, Riordan led her students through exploration of improvisation-based dance forms onto the level of dance performance as an art form. In San Francisco, the Prime Movers Company grew out of a recreational dance program for adults with intellectual disabilities (Hugill, 1992). Wolfgang Stange's professional dance company Amici in England includes members with and without intellectual disabilities. Touch Compass is New Zealand's first integrated dance company (Chappell, 2000), while in Australia people with intellectual disabilities perform in dance companies such as Restless Dance in Adelaide (Chance, 2000) and Company CHAOS from northern New South Wales (Worth, 2000). Benjamin (2001) documents the international reach of his work in improvisational performance with people with a range of disabilities in Making An Entrance. All of these options give people with intellectual disabilities and appropriate interest and talent, opportunities that are far beyond the scope of therapeutic or recreational dance.

How to select an appropriate dance form for clients with intellectual disabilities

It is clear that there are a number of possible alternatives for dance programs for people with intellectual disabilities, but not all of these are suitable for all individuals. The determining factors for choice of modality for a dance program with any group or individual are discussed below. They include:

⊚ the support needs of participants
⊚ their interest and ability in dance
⊚ the contract between group leader and participants
⊚ the skills and training of the group leader.

Level of clients' support needs

The aforementioned dance modalities can be seen as part of a continuum from dance therapy through to creative dance, community dance and to disability performance arts. The appropriateness of a particular modality for an individual client's needs is likely to be roughly equivalent to their support needs. Clients with higher support needs are usually better served by dance therapy, while those who function more independently usually have more to gain through a creative dance approach. Those individuals who are functioning at the most normal end of the IQ range might ideally be served by more mainstream recreational or community dance program. This continuum fits within the preferred paradigm of the least restrictive option for people with intellectual disabilities.

Clients' interest in and ability in dance

Another factor in the choice of appropriate dance modality is that of clients' interest in and talent for dance. This may or may not correspond with their support needs or abilities in other areas. Some high functioning clients may not be interested in the challenges of performing, while others with less competence in other areas may find dance performance a preferred expressive medium. Dance therapist Linda Murrow comments that 'individual level of ability/disability … does not correlate in any way with individual capacity for self-expression, creativity, wholeness, meaningful relationships, participation in a group or enjoyment of body movement' (1997, p. 2).

Contract between group leader and group/individual

As suggested by Morrish (1999), the contract between the group leader and the group/individual is an important determining factor in the choice of dance modality. The first priority in setting up dance programs for people with intellectual disabilities should be the establishment of a 'contract' with the host organisation, stating the purpose and desired outcomes of the program. These will be different in different situations, depending upon the organisation's purpose and the particular clientele.

For example, in one case a program was set up in an accommodation facility for independent adults with mild intellectual disabilities, because the recreation co-ordinator recognised the need for an after-work recreational activity that involved physical exercise. The program required the enrolment of a minimum number of adults who volunteered and paid for the activity themselves, so it had to be enjoyable. Therefore, the contract between the group leader and the host organisation on behalf of participants in this program was about recreation, fun and fitness. In this setting, the group leader needed the skills of a recreational dance teacher.

The focus of the dance program was quite different in a different type of facility. In a day centre for people with profound intellectual disabilities who had experienced life-long institutionalisation, the dance program needed a therapeutic focus. Clients' high support needs and very limited social skills made more basic goals appropriate. The contract between the group leader and this host organisation therefore was about the fostering of engagement, interaction and connection with others. The skills of a dance therapist were required for this program.

Practitioners' skills

A final consideration in the selection of an appropriate dance modality is that of the skills of the prospective group leader. Practitioners who have skills and training across the spectrum of the dance modalities discussed above will be able to offer varying programs to suit the different needs of client groups. Those whose skills are weighted towards one end or other of the spectrum will need to ensure that their skills match the needs of any prospective client group. Benjamin (2001), for example, whose background is professional dance, is very clear about his preference not to work with intellectually disabled participants who have challenging behaviours. He believes that his skills are best suited to the collaborative development of dance performance with people who have the capacity to contribute without assisted facilitation. He aspires to equality in his relationships with dance group participants. Dance therapists like Loman and Merman, on the other hand, are skilled in coping with the complex social, emotional and physical needs of their clients. They have less need, therefore, of well-developed choreographic and performance skills.

Making the right choice

Practitioners' responses to inappropriate selection of modalities are often described. My (Kim's) ambivalence about leading a performance-focused creative dance program in a special developmental school, is detailed in the following excerpt from the program diary:

> While there were many who seemed to really benefit from these new experiences, there were others for whom the group dance sessions seemed not to be particularly enjoyable or meaningful. Many of the more disabled students seemed to find the break in routine, noise and chaos (albeit controlled chaos) too much to cope with. One student, Luke, who was severely disabled with Down syndrome, sat out as far as he could from the group during every session, refusing to be involved in any way. Others, like Robert, who had autism, found that the physical contact required in dancing together was more than he could tolerate. He often withdrew to a corner of the room after activities that required him to touch or be touched by another student (1999a, p. 12).

I concluded that a therapeutic approach without any focus on performance outcome would have been much more beneficial for these low-functioning and socially isolated members of the school group.

On the other hand, practitioners who have as their intention the creation of professional performance get annoyed by the association of their work with therapy. Benjamin (2001) devotes a chapter of *Making An Entrance* to this issue. He describes his work as 'determinedly anti-therapeutic', in that it is 'about disabled and non-disabled people meeting of their own accord to improvise or perform together'.

Another model, one that he does not favour, is 'quasi-therapeutic dance', when people who are not disabled bring people with disabilities together and provide them with an experience of the arts. Benjamin does believe, however, that the experience of creating professional dance may have a clearly therapeutic effect, 'extending physical ability and improving self-esteem and confidence' (2001, p. 64). But this is not necessarily the case, and Benjamin acknowledges that with the wrong kind of leadership the experience of creating professional theatre may also be negative, confirming stereotypes and damaging self-esteem.

Melbourne-based theatre director Katrine Gabb is clear that the intention of her work with intellectually disabled members of her DVA group is the production of professional quality theatre. DVA's focus is not therapy or even community art, but rather theatre produced as a product for an outside audience. The company's intention is 'to make innovative and challenging (theatre) work' (Joy, 2002, p. 15).

Catherine Threlfall (2002) discusses a similar distinction with respect to the musical disciplines of music therapy and community music. She conceptualises the relationship of the two as concentric circles, with music therapy at the core, surrounded by community music, one aspect of which is disability arts.

Continuum: Dance therapy to creative dance to disability performing arts

It appears that there are a range of views about the value of dance therapy, creative dance and other modalities of dance for people with intellectual disabilities. Table 1.1 shows the continuum we recognise, listing the suitability of the various dance modalities for particular client populations, the focus and intended outcome of programs, and the skills required of a practitioner to lead these programs.

Table 1.1 DANCE MODALITIES AND THEIR SUITABILITY FOR DIFFERENT POPULATIONS OF PEOPLE WITH INTELLECTUAL DISABILITIES

Dance modality	Population for whom this is suitable	Program focus	Intended outcome	Practitioner's skills required (in order of priority)
Dance/ movement therapy	Clients with high support needs Clients with particularly challenging and/or antisocial behaviours	Therapeutic focus	Change within myself: Adjustment to society/ environment Development of relationship with others	DMT training Counselling and psychology skills required for a person-centred approach Motivation to serve clients' needs Group facilitation skills Laban-based movement skills

continued

Dance modality	Population for whom this is suitable	Program focus	Intended outcome	Practitioner's skills required (in order of priority)
Creative dance	Low/moderate/high functioning participants with recreational interest in dance	Recreational or educational focus	Enjoyment Experience valuable in itself Any change or development is a bonus Physical exercise	Extensive experience in movement and dance an advantage Group facilitation skills Basic choreographic skills Liaising skills: within group and people peripherally involved in program (parents, carers, etc)
Creative or community dance	Medium to high functioning clients with interest in performing	Dance for enjoyment Creating art with marginalised people Performance focus	Creative expressive opportunity for participants Developing a sense of community Political intention: challenging the status quo about what is art	Choreographic skills, ability to craft a piece for audience's pleasure Group facilitation skills Skills in advocacy for community arts Organisational and liaising skills: within group, general public, arts community, funding and government departments Ability to successfully conceptualise and obtain funding for a project
Disability arts as performance	High functioning and independent clients with vocational interest in performing arts	Skill development for individual and group Developing a group style Polished professional end product important	Can be art for arts sake Addressing social injustices Political intention: challenging the status quo about what is art	Sophisticated choreographic skills, ability to craft a piece for audience's pleasure Group facilitation skills Political motivation Artistic direction Understanding of theatre principles: design, lighting, presentation to audience Ability to successfully conceptualise and obtain funding for a project Organisational and liaising skills: within group, general public, arts community, funding and government departments

Chapter **2**

Creative dance using a Laban-based approach

The Laban framework

Rudolf Laban (1879–1958) was a pioneer in movement education and modern dance, and had a significant impact on the development of dance practice in the early to mid-twentieth century, initially in Europe and the United Kingdom. Later his thinking and writing influenced dance around the world, as the value of his framework in dance-related fields such as education, therapy, notation, research and choreography became manifest. Laban's work continues to this day at the Laban Centre in London, where training in dance, dance therapy and related disciplines are taught, and by numerous other institutions and practitioners whose activities have been informed by the Laban way of approaching dance and movement.

Marion North (1995, p. 6), a long-time scholar and teacher at the Centre, describes Laban's influence on the world of dance thus:

> Laban led the way in Europe against the confines of classical ballet … to create dance of a new and innovative kind – 'free dance' … genuinely freeing the body from the limitations of the ballet, imposed from outside, developed and refined over centuries. By breaking these restrictions he provided the opportunity for a range of new and expressive forms, limited only by the dancing individual's ability to 'soar free' and find new vocabulary. This was a genuinely new development for dance, which paralleled other innovations by pioneers in the USA. Instead of a set series of dance motifs and conventions, the whole range of human movement, and with it, the human emotions and inner life, became available to the choreographer and dancer.

Laban was interested in notions of expression and the individual. His concern was more with the process of creative exploration than what is evident in the performance for the audience. North describes how a deep link to the humanness of the dancer is created through Laban-based dance. 'It is not the doing of the activity which is important, but the linking of the inner being and the outer form' (1971, p. 23). The acknowledgement of the value of this process and the connection between the dance and the humanity of the dancer is what makes Laban's thinking about dance so significant.

Laban-based movement practice is different from most other dance styles in that it encourages the continuing expansion of a dancer's repertoire. This contrasts with the aesthetic framework of most other styles of dance that actually limit a participant's physical range. For example, classical ballet sanctions only light, graceful and upwards-focused movement for women, thereby reducing opportunities for experiences of groundedness and strength. The hands-in pocket style of country and western line dancing precludes any involvement of the arms and upper body. Dancing using only lower body and legs severely reduces opportunities for whole body integration, balance and co-ordination.

Schlusser describes how 'Laban movement concepts have been widely recognised for their value in working with people with special needs' (2000, p. 23), citing authors such as Leventhal (1982), Stinson (1990), Bond (1994), and Exiner and Kelynack (1994). Our experience has indicated the merit of the Laban framework's expressive and expansionist approach to movement and dance for people with intellectual disabilities. Movement restrictions imposed by physical and cognitive disabilities, and compounded by sedentary lifestyles and limited choices, make it particularly important that no further restrictions are placed on movement potential.

Dance program provides Robert with an opportunity to 'direct the traffic'

Robert was a 65-year-old man with slight cerebral palsy, some challenges with his balance, partial hearing impairment and a mild intellectual disability. He enjoyed coming to dance class for a number of years and was a very determined and co-operative class member, who would always do his utmost to participate in all class activities.

Robert's signature movement was a two-armed traffic policeman's wave. When students were asked to create a movement, as part of a warm-up, or during the creation of a choreography, Robert loved to do this wave and have the class emulate him, or perform it in canon, one member after another. Robert's dream in life was to have been a traffic director, and at BreakOut he often got his chance, an opportunity to direct the world in his own style.

As Laban investigated the underlying patterns and forms of human movement, he identified various aspects which together revealed the rich range of possible movement combinations. These concepts have since been expanded by many significant dance theorists to create a framework that is useful for describing, notating, evaluating, choreographing and teaching dance (including Bartenieff and Lewis, 1980; Bond, 1999; Dell, 1977; Moore and Yamamoto, 1988; and Stinson, 1988). The core concepts of this expanded framework that are useful for the purposes of this book are: Body, Space, Effort (Flow, Weight, Space and Time) and relationships, as outlined below.

Body: The 'What' of movement.
What is the body doing?

◎ *Body part functions:*
  - What part/s of the body is/are moving?
  - Where is the movement initiated? (from the centre, from the periphery of the body?)
  - Does a body part consistently lead movement, or is it consistently held or inert?
  - Are body parts in use simultaneously or sequentially?

◎ *Body actions:* What kind of movement is going on?
  (e.g. walk, run, skip, jump, tiptoe, leap, stamp?)

◎ *Body shape*: What shape does the body make? How is it held?

Space: The 'Where' of movement.
Where is the body moving?

◎ *Direction:* Where does the body, or the movement travel?
  (e.g. forward, backwards, sideways, up, down?)

◎ *Size:* How large or small are the movements?

◎ *Pathways*: What is the pattern the body makes as it travels
  through the air or on the floor?
  (e.g. straight, curved, zig-zag, spiral, twisted?)

◎ *Level:* What level is the movement? (the vertical distance from the floor)
  High, medium or low?

◎ *Focus:* Where do the eyes look?
  (e.g. straight ahead, to the corner, to the side, towards a partner, to the other side of the space?)

◎ *Dimensions:* One-dimensional movement: horizontal, vertical and sagittal axes
  - Horizontal axis (does the body move sideways/across?)
  - Vertical axis (does the body move upward/downward?)
  - Sagittal axis (does the body move forward/backward?)

◎ *Planes:* Two-dimensional movement:
  - Door plane (vertical and horizontal movement)
  - Table (horizontal and sagittal movement)
  - Wheel plane (sagittal and vertical movement)
  - Vertical plane: related to presentation of oneself
  - Horizontal plane: related to communication with others
  - Sagittal plane: related to decision/operation/action

◎ *Three-dimensional movement:* spirals, diagonals, cubes

Effort: The 'How' of movement.
How is the body moving?

This aspect of movement is concerned with the amount of energy used and how it is released. Effort comprises four elements: Flow, Weight, Space and Time.

Flow

Flow has to do with how ongoing the movement is, on a continuum from bound to free flow.

◎　*Bound flow:* When energy is released in a controlled, restrained way, so movement could readily stop. This is the feeling you might have if you were trying to place a precious vase on a high shelf.

◎　*Free flow:* When energy is released freely, the feeling you might have if you were dancing with abandon to a favourite piece of music.

Weight

Weight is about the continuum of strength to lightness.

◎　*Strong weight:* The feeling you would have if you were trying to squash a cockroach with your foot.

◎　*Light weight:* The feeling you might have if you were trying to walk past someone sleeping without being heard.

◎　A third possibility is *heavy weight:* A passive feeling. In Laban terms, heavy is not the opposite to lightness, but rather an absence of energy. It is the feeling you would have if you were lying completely relaxed on the floor.

Space

Space is about the continuum of direct and indirect movement intention.

◎　*Direct:* would be the way you might travel if you saw someone on the other side of the street and were trying to make your way straight to them.

◎　*Indirect:* would be the way you might travel if you were window-shopping without a particular destination or time limitation.

Time

Time is about the relationship of one movement or part of a movement to another.

◎　*Sudden/sustained:* The speed of movement refers to how slow or fast it is. In Laban terminology, time is defined on the continuum of suddenness to sustainment, thereby describing the quality of time associated with a movement rather than an actual period of time a movement may take.

◎　*Duration:* The length of time movement lasts; a long time, a short time, or something in between. Duration is often but not always related to speed. (You can move slowly for a long time, or quickly for a short time.)

◎　*Phrase:* Longer sequences of movement that have a sense of completeness by themselves. A phrase can be thought of as a 'dance sentence'. An example might be: Walk and reach and touch and stop …

Relationship: relationships created through movement

◎ *Relationships:* between body parts, different movements and shapes, individuals and groups, as well as with the environment. Some of these concepts are:

- towards and away from
- around
- through
- between
- over and under
- before and after
- faster and slower
- alike and different.

◎ *Relationship of body parts:* the way parts of the body relate to each other. For example:

- the line between head, neck and shoulders
- the way the arms are positioned in relation to the torso.

◎ *Relationships between people:* ways one person relates to another or others through movement. Activities that could be used to explore interpersonal relationships through movement might be:

- finding a way to connect with another person using your hands, or using no hands
- moving with a partner without touching.
- travelling together as a group.

◎ *Relationship with objects:* props can be useful as a way of exploring another dimension of relationship. For example, a long flowing piece of fabric might offer improvisational opportunities for moving under, over, around, between and through.

LMA: Laban Movement Analysis

Laban's framework also included the development of a language for observing and describing human movement based on the aforementioned principles, that is now known as LMA (Laban Movement Analysis). LMA has many and varied applications, but in the context of dance practice with people who have disabilities, it can be useful as a tool for movement observation by teachers, therapists and group leaders. It can supplement the assessment and treatment of physical and other imbalances and as a choreographic aid. Bond (1999) describes the value of LMA thus: 'By making it possible to understand one of major vehicles of human meaning, namely movement, LMA can play a significant role in the evolution of human learning'. More about the use of LMA as an evaluative tool appears in Chapter 10 on Evaluation.

The art of improvisation

Since the early twentieth century, when Laban began his influential work, there has been much development in dance practice that goes beyond codified technique, expanding possibilities for the art form and for artists. Fran Levy describes a movement active in the early twentieth century, not only in the arts, but in politics and society at large, to 'liberate the person, and to examine the full range of human behaviour and the motivation behind it' (1988, p. 2). The dance form of improvisation developed at this time, pioneered by people such as Isadora Duncan, whose expressive dance form was inspired by classical Greek theatre. Her unique contribution is referred to by dance therapist Claire Schmais:

> [Duncan was] the first to break away from the stultifying structure of classical ballet and champion dance as the emanation of emotions in harmony with the external forces of the natural world. She saw dance as man's most fundamental response to the universe; reviving man's capacity to dance was the means through which his ability to live fully and freely could be renewed (1974, pp. 7–8).

Duncan's work was a precursor to many contemporary modern and creative dancers, innovators like Ruth St Denis and Ted Shawn in America, and Mary Wigman in Germany.

The modern dance movement of the early 1900s also formed the basis of dance therapy. The experiences of teaching and performing led modern dancers such as Mary Whitehouse, Franziska Boas and Liljian Espenak, and later Trudi Schoop and Irmgard Bartenieff, 'to recognize the potential benefits of dance and movement as a form of psychotherapy' (Levy 1988, p. 2).

The art of improvisation as it is practised in the twenty-first century developed out of modern dance. Improvisation is about opening up to impulse and tapping into the subconscious without intellectual censorship. Improvisation allows spontaneous and simultaneous exploration, creation and performance (Blom and Chaplin 1988, p. ix). Nachmanovitch describes it as 'the master key to creativity'(1990, p. 9).

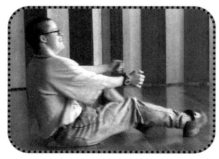

Improvised dance is particularly valuable for people with intellectual disabilities because it requires less memory (cognitive and muscle) than most other dance forms and can accommodate diverse body shapes and abilities. In improvised dance, participants and the audience appreciate the shapes and movements created spontaneously in response to the energy and mood of the group. They can be surprised and delighted by what is different and unique, rather than thinking of difference in terms of imperfections, mistakes or an absence of skills. For these reasons, improvisation is the basis for much of our work with people who have intellectual disabilities.

In the next section we discuss issues about decision-making for program planning; how a group leader decides what dance form is most appropriate for participants.

Structuring the session: Improvisation versus technique

In preparing sessions, a dance group leader can think of working on a continuum from prescriptive to more open and improvised movement. There are times when improvisation will be the best strategy for developing a session, enabling a flow from beginning to end that more structured material won't allow. The freedom of improvisation means that there can be a focus on process rather than outcome. It also eliminates the feeling of defeat that can be experienced by participants and the group leader if a particular form is not achieved. When working with people who have severe disabilities there is often very little obvious response and engagement. In this situation, any desire to teach a structured form of dance needs to be put to one side.

Improvisation is also about freeing up movement when it has become locked into a particular pattern or style. Having the opportunity to move freely will benefit those participants who have only experienced dancing in a set style, such as line dancing, rock'n'roll or jazz ballet. Through improvisation, participants might discover and enjoy another movement quality not present in the techniques of dance styles they have previously learned. Improvisation can also be beneficial for those people whose movement vocabulary is limited by their disability. For example, some people with Down syndrome have a preference for heavy, slow movement. Through playing with improvised movement in a dance session they can experience another way of moving, perhaps using lightness, strength and quickness.

Melissa experiences strength through elastic stretching activity

BreakOut member Melissa is a large woman with Down syndrome, who moves with great fluidity and slow languor. Sometimes she appears exhausted. However, Melissa can stretch her body with great ease and is full of creative ideas. One day in class she was given a piece of elastic to hold and stretch, in an activity designed for participants to experiment with the feeling of strength and bound flow. Melissa found it very difficult to grip the elastic with enough strength to hold it. When she was asked to extend it out as far as she could before letting it go she was barely able to pull it any wider than its resting length and sat holding it limply.

When the same activity was repeated in the next session, Melissa displayed more confidence in handling the elastic. She held it firmly and then found she could stretch it. As she pulled the elastic wide, Melissa began to make different shapes. She drew on strength that she hadn't been able to access the week before. The experience of improvising with the elastic had led Melissa to an uncharacteristic movement expression that incorporated strength and bound flow.

Improvisation will also benefit those people whose exposure to any creative process has been limited. It is about creating an environment in which self-expression is valued and encouraged.

The impact of creative dance experience

One day as I (Kim) started work with a new group, I began as I generally do in any BreakOut session but found that this time the outcome was very different. I was accustomed to introducing the ritual warm-up activity of 'make your own move' and then to have members vigorously and enthusiastically create their own movements and model them for the class to follow. When I asked these new participants to create their own movements they responded with bewilderment, not understanding what I wanted them to do. I realised that the process of creating one's own movement needed to be modelled by me and then practised before new dancers could confidently tackle the challenge.

Later, I reflected on how much BreakOut members have developed as a result of participation in a creative movement process. The skills they have acquired through regular practice include expansion of movement repertoire and increased confidence to perform and lead a group. This observation was confirmed by a visiting dance student, who commented on BreakOut members' rich and idiosyncratic movement repertoires and ability to take the lead during sessions.

With groups who need to develop skills in co-operating and functioning as a community, more structured activities may be desirable. While it is important for people to be able to express their individuality through the creative possibilities of dance, it is also important that they are able to work together, to co-operate and create a shared experience. Many people with poor communication skills and those with autism find this challenging. Through dance, however, they may be able to find an enjoyable vehicle for achieving participation, a means of communication and a way of experiencing non-demanding physical touch.

The challenge for a group leader is to know when to choose an improvisational mode of working, and when a more structured mode would be most beneficial. While the rest of this chapter describes activities that are based on a Laban framework, and include improvised elements, there are many enjoyable dance activities that are based on more structured style, including folk or social dancing. These can help establish focus in a group, draw participants together and develop group co-operation. More specific information about folk and popular dance can be found in Chapter 5.

It can also be beneficial to work towards a performance, as a way of marking the group's achievement and to provide a focus for activities. This process is discussed in Chapter 6, and includes ideas for creating performances of different kinds, as well as models for performance and outcomes.

Fitness through dance

In addition to creative expression, a dance program can also make a contribution to participants' physical fitness. Stamina, strength and stretch, known as the three Ss, are the main principles of fitness. A creative dance program has the capacity to contribute to participants' fitness in all three areas.

Stamina

Stamina refers to the cardiovascular component of an activity. It is improved by aerobic exercise, which means breathing in air to supply oxygen continuously to working muscles. Aerobic fitness is developed and maintained through large muscle activities that allow sustained metabolism. The benefits of aerobic exercise are many, including:

- improved circulation, respiration and fat metabolism
- reduced stress levels, body fat and risk of heart disease
- stronger bones, ligaments and tendons
- weight control
- more energy and less fatigue
- enhanced mood, self-concept and body image
- greater emotional stability
- a more positive outlook (Sharkey, 1990).

Strength

Strength can be defined as the maximum force that can be exerted in a single voluntary contraction. It assists with improving posture and overall body shape. Phasic muscles, those that are more active when we are in motion, such as quadriceps (thigh muscles), abdominals and tibialis anterior (shins) and pectorals (chest) in the upper limb, tend to weaken and lose tone with age, especially if they are relaxed too often. They need strengthening to reduce loss of tone, and to reduce fat accumulations that occur with age.

Suppleness or stretch

This is the range of motion through which the limbs are able to move, and is attained through stretching. This is one of the most important aspects of fitness, as it is necessary to improve general flexibility and avoid injury.

Stretching is vital because the postural muscles, such as calves, hamstrings, back extensors, iliopsoas (hip flexors) and deep back muscles that support us when we stand, sit and lie down, tend to tighten when they are not used.

How to stretch

The most effective static stretching involves using slow movements to reach a point of stretch, holding the position for five to ten seconds and relaxing. Another method is the contract–relax technique, which begins with a static stretch, then relaxing, contracting the muscle briefly, then repeating the static stretch (St.George, 1994).

Musical accompaniment

There are suggestions for accompanying music listed with each of the activities described below. This assumes that the dance group does not have live musicians available to accompany the session. Any opportunity of accompaniment by live music should be welcomed, as it offers the additional dimensions of life, energy and variations that come from music made by real people rather than machines. In Chapter 5 (page 128) we recall a workshop that involved live drumming and explain how this was incorporated into a dance session and performance. Group leaders should also explore possibilities of activities performed in silence, or with the accompaniment of voice and/or percussion instruments.

Elements of a creative dance session

The rest of this chapter describes the framework for sessions we have developed and recommended activities. The list is by no means exhaustive, but is a good starting point for activities that can be used successfully in dance programs for people with intellectual disabilities. The program we outline aims to encourage the expression of the humanity of the person, rather than any particular form or movement. Opportunities for participants to create their own movement ideas are recommended.

Elements of a creative dance session

- **Warm-up**
- **Stretch and strengthen**
- **Theme: the body of the session**
- **Improvisation and solos**
- **Relaxation**
- **Closure.**

A lesson may include any or all of these elements. A good warm-up and a ritual closure are really important so that all participants are clear about the beginning and end of the session.

Warm-up

A warm-up prepares group members for the activities to come, both physically and psychologically. In classes for people with intellectual disabilities we almost always warm up in a circle. This is a way of including all members, ensuring eye contact between individuals and the whole class and making sure everyone has all the cues they can to follow. In a circle everyone can see and hear each other, so vocal cues can be used when a participant's vision is not so good. Those who are less tuned in to verbal communication have a good view of the leader and the group. The energy flow of a circle functions to hold the group together as well.

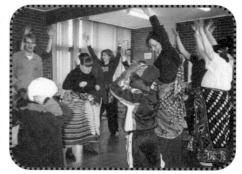

Circle power!

The power of a circle was demonstrated in the opening dance of a performance by BreakOut. The choreography for this piece was based on a circular design. A circle of fabric on the floor was encircled by a ring of chairs on which the dancers (all older adults with mild to moderate intellectual disabilities) were positioned. As the performance began, one member of this group decided not to continue with the planned item, but to draw attention to herself instead by staying outside the circle and making loud and inappropriate verbal comments. Performers, staff and participants, all did their best to ignore Debbie and to involve themselves totally in the performance experience that included drum rhythms, the manipulation of the giant coloured fabric circle and slow mesmerising wave-like movements. Eventually she tired of being on the outside, especially since she appeared to be having little impact on the attention of the performers, and was drawn into the more powerful energy of the circle. The item finished with all members, including Debbie, being totally absorbed in what they were doing.

Following are five suggested activities for a warm-up.

Welcome

Aims

Finding a way to welcome participants to the session is an important starting point. This is about acknowledging each person's presence, helping them feel at ease and facilitating the transition into the dance session. Once a group is established they will probably feel at home with a particular greeting and look forward to it. The welcome becomes a ritual in which participants and group leader alike enjoy the ease and familiarity of coming together for another session. Listed below are some suggestions for ways of welcoming groups.

◉   *Eye contact:* The leader begins by walking around the circle, making eye contact and saying hello. If the group or an individual is non-verbal, the leader needs to look carefully for their response. In one of the groups I (Jenny) lead, I am greeted by a diversity of non-verbal responses: a smile, eye blinking, a movement of the hand, vocalising, a handshake, a forward movement of the head. Over the years of being with this group these responses have become significant in my understanding and valuing of each individual.

◉   *Handshake:* The leader walks around the circle and extends their hand for a handshake. This is more direct approach. The leader will need to establish whether the person feels comfortable with you entering their personal space in this way. Try eye contact first. If a person cannot unfold their hand, a light brush across the surface of the hand is an alternative approach. Hand contact is also a good means of establishing contact with people who have visual and hearing impairments.

◎   *Name song:* There are a number of simple greeting songs that involve moving around the circle and singing each person's name. For example,
'*Who's in the circle today?*' It goes like this:
'*Who's in the circle today, today, who's in the circle today?*'
'***Name*** *is in the circle today, today and* ***Name*** *is in the circle today.*'
Wait for a response and then continue moving to the next person in the circle.
'***Name*** *is in the circle today, today, and* ***Name*** *is in the circle today.*'
Wait for a response and continue singing the line above, moving onto the next person in the circle. Accompany the singing with clapping to a steady beat.
This can also be sung without waiting for responses so that the clapping is continuous and the song builds up momentum as it moves around the circle.

◎   *Name and movement:* This is a good one to do when you are meeting a group for the first time. It requires group members to have some degree of confidence in their own movement and expressing themselves in front of a group. Start by standing or sitting in a circle. One person starts by saying their name and simultaneously making a movement. The group leader could model this to begin with. The group watches and then everyone together repeats the person's name and movement. Progress around the circle, moving either clockwise or anti-clockwise.

Teaching Tip: The 3 Rs – rhythm, repetition and ritual

An effective means of bringing focus to a group is by setting up a strong rhythm, either by clapping, stamping and/or vocalising and then repeating it. The song 'Who's in the circle today?' is a good example. When this song is repeated week after week so that it becomes part of the ritual of the session, the group will enter into the power of the rhythm and their attention will be focused from the very beginning. Less energy will need to be expended by the group leader to draw individuals into the action after such an activity.

Swapping chairs

Aims
Focusing, co-operation, decision making, gentle exercise.

Description
Participants sit on chairs in a circle all facing the centre. Group leader takes out his/her chair so that there is one less chair than the number of participants. She/he then begins the activity by walking across the circle to tap another participant on the shoulder. This indicates to that person they must give up their chair and choose another. The chosen person continues the activity by standing up and walking across the circle to make their choice. The game continues until the group leader returns the extra chair to the circle.

Variations

◉ The person who is walking across the circle balances a bean-bag on their head. Instead of tapping the chosen person on their shoulder, they allow the bean-bag to slide from their head into the chosen person's lap.

◉ The person moving can create their own movements as they travel across the circle using their own individual movement style.

Music

No music necessary.

Simple circle walking

Aims

Warm-up of major muscle groups, co-ordination, stimulation of thinking, new patterns of movement, direction, spatial orientation, co-operation, listening and following instructions.

Description

Walking on the spot, all facing in. This gives the class a chance to see each other, to say hello, and ensures that everyone in the group can be in the leader's line of vision. Knees lift up and down in the walk, warming the large muscle groups in the legs and buttocks. This will also get energy flowing through people's bodies.

Variations

There are unlimited possibilities with this – a different beginning for every class, based on a similar formula. Some of these are listed below.

◉ *Walking in and out of the circle:* The group stands in a circle holding hands, walking into and away from the centre of the circle. This is ideal to begin with as it is very inclusive and the rhythm encourages all class members to work at more or less the same pace. It is also the best way to include those who tend to daydream or wander off. It can be difficult to get a group moving together in a circle, but once this skill is mastered many other activities will be much easier.

◉ *Moving to the centre*
  • Call out a greeting when you reach the centre: *Hello, g'day, good morning*
  • Two people at a time move to the centre and greet each other with a *Hi 5* (one palm clapped with the partner's), or *Give Me 10*, (both palms to partner's palms)
  • Arms go up as the group moves towards the centre and down again as the group goes out.
  • Divide the group, some going in while others stay out. For example, the leader might call out, 'Women all in, men stay where they are'. This can create some hilarity when people aren't too sure who is which, but others can offer their opinions.
  • Try other ways to divide up the group and get people thinking – by clothing, e.g. all those with T-shirts on, all those with bare feet, all those wearing red.
    Providing variations like these can assist group members to identify themselves as separate and different individuals from others in the group.

◉ *Changing directions:* Backwards and sideways – try walking in and out backwards or sideways for a different challenge.

⊚ *Varying levels:* Low, medium or high – vary the level at which you are working. Members might bend down low as they walk, or stretch right up high.

⊚ *Varying energy:* Try experimenting with different weight qualities, for example, strength expressed through stamps and jumps, or lightness expressed through gentle steps or walking on tiptoe.

⊚ *Travelling around the circle:* The circle can travel clockwise or anti-clockwise. It doesn't hurt to offer this instruction, but most of your clients and probably your staff will need you to demonstrate the direction. You can change direction slowly at first, but do it faster as people master the concept and the skills required to change (i.e. stop, turn, re-negotiate changing hands and reconnecting, re-propel in the opposite direction).

Music

Lively music with a strong regular beat and medium tempo is best. The ideal is a recording that has suitable tracks following each other, so that the session is not disrupted by the leader having to change CDs. Some ideas:

⊚ Thula Sana, *Thula Sana*, or other African music with a steady beat and infectious rhythm

⊚ Tribal Trance, *Minjarah* – a slightly faster beat that gets people moving.

⊚ Kylie Minogue, *Light Years 2000* - familiar pop songs.

Teaching Tip: What to do if the circle isn't happening!

Not every group will form a circle with ease. The need for personal space, the long-term effect of disassociation, the unfamiliarity of the experience and difficulty in understanding an abstract concept could all be contributing factors to the challenge for some groups.

To help develop a circle it is a good idea to start with marking it out in some way. Chairs are very effective. Place a circle of chairs in the centre of the room for people to sit on when they enter the session. If you want to start with participants standing up, mark out a circle with masking tape and decorate it with the colours of the rainbow. Group members can choose their favourite colour to stand on. At first you may be the only person standing or sitting in the circle. Some behaviours take a lifetime to form and won't change overnight, so don't be discouraged!

You may have to move away from the circle after the initial welcoming time and meet people where they have positioned themselves in the room. However, starting and finishing in the circle will help establish the pattern. With repetition will come familiarity and one day you just might find yourself standing in a circle with the whole class holding hands!

Pairing up

Aims

Continues warm-up as for 2, adding the complexity of co-operation with another person through a variety of partnering combinations

Description

There are hundreds of different ways that two people can move together as partners. Here are a few ideas. No doubt your group can think of more of their own.

Music

The dynamics of movement elicited will depend on the dynamic quality of the music you use. Music of a particular genre will elicit qualities of movement appropriate for that style. Some suggestions for movement-inspiring music are given below.

Variations

◎   Place hands on each others shoulders and spin, clockwise and anti-clockwise.

◎   Stand back to back and circle together, clockwise and anti-clockwise.

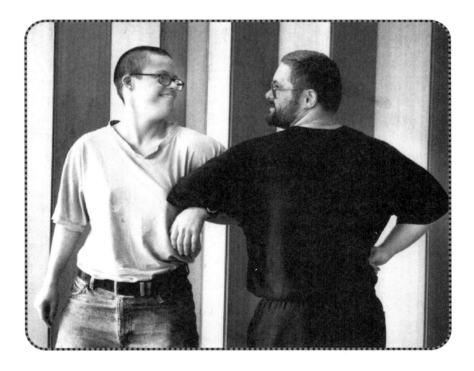

◎   *Bush dance style 'arming':* partners link right elbows to circle clockwise, then change elbows to circle anti-clockwise.
Music suggestion: Bush dance music such as 'Morrison's Jig' and 'The Brown Jug Polka' from Shenanigans, *International Bush Dancing*.

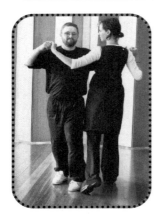

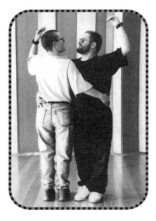

⊚ *Swing dance style:* partners face each other holding hands, stepping in towards each other and back, arms opening wide as you step in.

Music suggestion: rock'n'roll compilations such as *Hooked On Rock'n'Roll*

⊚ *Israeli style:* Partners stand together, touching right hip to right hip, facing in opposite directions. Right arm goes around the front of partner's body to hold their waist, and left arm is held up high. Heads turn in to look in to each other. This is a great position for a fast swing. Change body direction, hips and arms to travel the other way.

Music suggestion: Israeli or Klezmer music such as 'Dancing On Water', 'Meron Nign' from *A Jewish Odyssey* or Klezmania's *Oystralia*

⊚ *Do-si-do square dance style:* Partners face each other about 1 metre apart. Walk towards each other, then pass right shoulders, cross back to back and return to original position without changing body direction.

Music suggestion: Country dance music like Shania Twain, *Shania Twain*, or *Line Dance: The Ultimate Collection*.

⊚ *Rock'n'roll style twist and turn:* Partners extend right hand like a handshake to their partner, then step back slightly to extend arms. Turn to face clockwise and use small twisting movements of the lower body to travel around in a circle.

Music suggestion: Elvis Presley, *Presley*, or *The Best Ever Disco Album*.

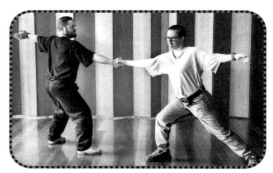

⊚ *Changing partners.* Begin with class members pairing up with a friend. These two dance together for a few minutes, then move on to a new partner. The group could keep changing partners, like you might in a progressive barn dance, or the group leader might give the group more specific instructions like:
'Find a new partner, someone you haven't been with today.'
'Find someone you don't know very well.'
'Men, find a woman partner; ladies, find a man to work with.'

Knee bounces

Aims
Whole body integration, stretch and release.

Description
Stand with feet comfortably hip-width apart. Relax knees and ankles, arms hang by your sides. Get a rhythm going through the body, by bending and stretching the knees to make a gentle bounce, with arms swinging by the sides.

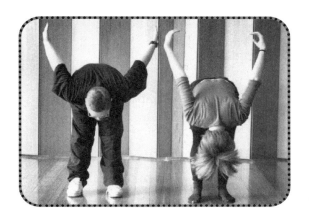

Make a short phrase by adding an ending to a series of bounces:

- the body drops forward over the knees
- the body lifts up high at the end of a phrase
- the body swings to the side
- the body twists to the side.

Variations
- Arms can swing close to the body or high
- Arms can swing right up overhead, lifting the body up into a balance
- Arms can swing in opposition (one goes forward while the other swings backwards–challenging!)
- Arms can also swing side to side, leading the body into a twist or a tilt, giving the torso a stretch.
- Class members can create their own body shape at the end of a phrase.

Music
Words can help members keep the rhythm, such as:

Bounce and bounce and bounce and drop … bounce and bounce and bounce and lift, bounce and bounce and bounce and twist, bounce and bounce and bounce and bend.

Music in 3/4 time, including country and western style ballads is good for this kind of activity such as:

- Tammy Wynette, 'Lucille' and 'Singing My Song', *Country Music Giants*
- Aretha Franklin, 'Spanish Harlem', *Best of Aretha Franklin*
- Christine Anu , 'Island Home', *Stylin' Up.*

Safe dance tip: Keep a soft bend in the knee

Encourage the group to keep their knees gently flexed throughout warm-up activities. This takes the pressure off the lower back and acts as a cushion for joints and the spine, absorbing shock from vigorous movement.

Make your own move

Aims

This activity offers participants the opportunity to enjoy their own preferred movement style and have that affirmed by others. It also offers opportunities for all members to try new moves.

Description

This part of the warm-up at BreakOut has become a popular ritual. Class members begin each session by enthusiastically contributing their own ideas, new ideas as well as old favourites or movement signatures. If the class has done some circle walking or other simple locomotor movement for approximately 10 minutes by this time, then any move is pretty safe. Otherwise, begin with smaller, gentler movements to ensure that participants and staff are warm enough to prevent muscle injury. The leader might take the first turn and set the pace with a small, gentle movement.

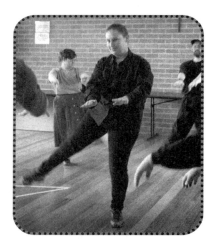

Safe dance tip: Work from the feet up and from big to small muscle groups.

In the warm-up, always begin with the larger muscle groups and work to the smaller, e.g. focus on legs before feet, feet before toes. Work from the bottom of the body up, i.e. focus on lower half of the body before upper half. This means movements of head and neck should be last, ensuring that the blood is flowing well before more vulnerable parts of the body are moved.

Variations

Anything is possible, but some simple ones include:

◎ *Heels touch:* Extend right leg forward, heel to the floor, then bring feet together before repeating with left heel. This assists with ability to change weight, identify right and left, articulate feet, especially heels, and lengthen Achilles tendon and calf muscles.

◎ *Toes touch:* Same again, but touching toes to the floor, giving a stretch to the toes and top of the foot.

◎ *Steps to the side* (right and left) with an arm action, e.g. step and clap or step and click.

◎ *Double step to the side* (step to right, bring feet together, step to right, bring feet together again; repeat all to the left side).

◎ *Jumps:* Star jumps, jack-jumps, bounces on the spot (not everyone will be delighted about this one, but you don't have to do too many).

◎ *Reach and stretch:* Stretch to the side, forward or behind, reaching out with arms, as if you wanted to grab something but your feet are stuck on the spot. Keep a gentle bend in the knee.

◎ *Squats:* Bend down to touch the floor. (Take this slowly, especially for older and heavier participants. Avoid it if it hurts. Deep knee bends below 90 degrees should be avoided.)

◎ *Swings:* Swing the torso around from side to side, wrapping your arms around your body as you go. It is important for knees to be gently flexed in this one. Look over each shoulder as you go from side to side, and encourage participants to think about their heads as part of their body and use the full length of their spine.

◎ *Kicks:* Kicking legs up alternately. Experiment with different directions to kick, e.g. sideways and backwards.

◎ *Turns:* Some participants, especially those with autism, may particularly enjoy turning or spinning. Others will find it more difficult, especially those with cerebral palsy or other co-ordination challenges. It is always beneficial extending class members' repertoire with non-preferred movement actions.

Julia's lively warm-up moves

One student who really enjoys this part of the session at BreakOut is Julia, a very lively young woman with Down syndrome. The warm-up gives Julia an outlet for her rambunctious energy. She loves to go wild in movement surrounded by an affirming circle of BreakOut members. The rest of the group are not always so enthusiastic about

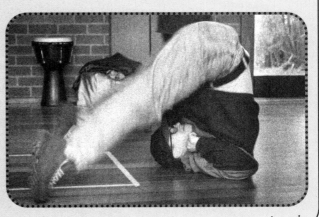

continued

Julia's moves, especially when she does her favourite move, a spinning roll on her back on the floor, followed by a backward somersault, a jump up and a series of duck hops on one leg, while turning in a circle. The more sedate group members and staff members on less energetic days don't necessarily follow Julia's moves exactly, but everyone is inspired by her energy and free flowing movement.

Safe dance tip: Encourage people to work within their own limits.

Support them to have the courage to try something new. Trying something new is commendable and to be encouraged but participants should feel free to stop when they have had enough. Some group members will have spent much of their lives doing what they are told and will feel obliged to please a leader by doing exactly what has been asked or demonstrated, even if it is beyond their capability or comfort zone. Others have adjusted to difficult circumstances by avoiding change and new challenges, and will face each new challenge with the view that they don't want to try it. Encourage these people to take it slowly. They might like to watch for quite some time before they try something new themselves.

Stretch and strengthen

Stretching and strengthening activities are vital aspects of fitness. For people with high muscle tone, activities to stretch and lengthen muscles are really important. For many people with Down syndrome who have low muscle tone and hypermobility, activities that result in increased muscle strength are a priority.

Safe dance tip: General guidelines for stretching
- Hold all stretches for a minimum of 6–10 seconds.
- Relax and breathe out as you move into the stretch.
- Push to the point of discomfort but do not push through pain.
- People with more serious physical disabilities, such as cerebral palsy, may need a different approach. Muscle contraction before release could be a more appropriate movement process. We recommend that advice from participants' physiotherapist be sought prior to commencement of a dance program.
- No exercise should cause pain.

The following activities have been modified for simplicity from those recommended for general fitness programs. They have been ordered so that the body is worked through in sequence and to make the minimum number of position changes, which can be time-consuming. Verbal instructions as they might be given to a group appear below, including some simple imagery that can help participants attain the feeling of a movement. The most effective teaching strategies are likely to be demonstration by the group leader or assistant and tactile cues (i.e. actually physically helping participants make the positions).

Allow participants time to position themselves. For some people, the idea of identifying a particular body part and manipulating it in a particular way will be a new experience.

Older adults, or those with more physical restrictions, may find it more beneficial to stretch supported by a chair. Modified exercises for people who prefer to remain seated are listed in Chapter 4 (page 95).

The ideal time for stretching is after the warm-up, so that participants' muscles are warm, with plenty of aerated blood flow. It is not necessary to incorporate all of these exercises in every session or even essential that every session includes a stretch and strengthen component. However, if participants are not physically extending themselves in your dance program, they are unlikely to be doing it elsewhere.

A focus of the stretch segment for a session might be a specific area of the body, perhaps an area that is likely to be in heavy use that day. For example, if the planned activities are going to include lots of arm movements, then exercises for arm stretching and strengthening are helpful.

The end of the session is another time when stretching should be included, if participants have been doing activities that are particularly demanding on any part of the body. For example, if the session has included a lot of high impact activities such as jumping, then exercises to stretch out the muscles in the thighs, shins and calves should be incorporated into the cool-down at the end of the session.

Following are half a dozen suggested streching activities.

Neck exercises (standing or sitting)

Neck flexion
Tuck your chin in and drop your head forward as if you want to see your knees.

Neck extension
Look to the ceiling and stretch your neck backwards. Make your muscles long as you gently tilt your head back.

Neck rotation
Look over one shoulder as far as you can, then turn to the other side.

Neck side flexion.
Let your head tilt down towards your shoulder. Now try it to the other shoulder.

Back, shoulder and chest exercises (standing or sitting)

Overhead stretch
Hold your own hands together, then reach up over your head to make a shape like a long pencil. Then gently stretch your arms back behind your head. Now let your hands go and reach down to see if you can touch the back of your neck. Can you make your elbows open wide?

Shoulder rotations for mobility
Can you make a circle with your shoulders? Try rolling them forwards, up and back. Now try it the opposite way, going backwards first.

Shoulder shrugs to release shoulder tension
Lift both shoulders up to your ears. Make the muscles in your shoulder and neck tight, then release them, as if you were saying, 'I don't know'.

Back stretch with flexed legs
Stand tall with your feet apart as wide as your hips. Bend your knees a little, then slowly bend over, reaching forward to touch the ground near your feet. Hold for a minute, then take a deep breath in and pull in the muscles in your stomach to help you slowly come up to standing position.

Side bends to lengthen muscles in the waist and torso
Keeping your knees slightly bent, stretch one arm overhead and put the other hand on your hip. Slowly bend to the side as if you wanted to reach out and touch the person next to you. Bob gently. Then come back to the centre and try it to the other side.

Side twist to lengthen muscles in the waist and torso
Stand with your feet comfortably apart and stretch your arms out wide to the side. Twist around to look at the person next to you. Come back to the centre and try it to the other side.

Elbow thrusts for shoulder and back
Stand with your feet comfortably apart. Put your hands on your shoulders and lift your elbows up in front of you. Then open your elbows out wide to the side. Now see if you can press your elbows back behind your body, then bring them slowly forward to touch them together.

Floor exercises for back, spine, buttocks, hips, thighs and hamstrings

Hamstring stretch
Sit on the floor with your legs stretched out in front of your body. Pull your toes towards you. Feel the stretch in your shin muscles.

Seated toe stretch for back and hamstrings
Stretch out your toes, then slowly slide your hands down your legs, letting your body drop forward until you feel a stretch. Hold your body in that position. Can you reach your hands down to your ankles? Hold it for a minute, then relax. Pull your toes back towards you and see if you can touch them.

Lower back stretch

Sit with one leg stretched out in front of you. Put your other foot against the thigh of the leg that is stretched out and let the knee drop down to the floor. Reach towards the toe you have stretched out, keeping your neck and shoulders relaxed. Feel the stretch all the way from the lower part of the back.

Hip stretch

Sitting with your legs crossed, gently reach forward with your body so that your arms touch the floor. Can you get your elbows down to the floor? Slowly slide back up again to your sitting position. Now stretch forward again, but slide a little to the left to feel all the muscles in your hips stretch. Slide back up to the centre before you try it again to the right.

Try the whole thing again with your legs crossed the opposite way.

Ankle pull for groin and inner thigh

Sit with the soles of your feet together. Hold your ankles with your hands while you gently press your legs down towards the floor with your elbows. Then lean forward and try to touch the floor with your head.

On all fours

Cat arch mobility exercise for the spine

Breathe in as you let your spine contract and curl inwards, breathe out as you arch your spine. Imagine you are a cat stretching after a big drink of milk.

Lower back release

Kneel on floor, sitting with your bottom positioned back on your ankles. Gradually drop your body forward over your knees and reach your arms forward along the floor.

Lying on stomach on the floor

Passive back arch and abdominal stretch.

Lie flat on the floor, with your hands flat on the floor beside your shoulders and your elbows close to your body. Breathe in and then gently push your body up from the floor. Keep your hips and legs on the floor. Try to keep your spine and neck long.

Modified push-ups to strengthen chest and upper arms

Lie flat with palms on the floor beside your shoulders, with your legs bent up at the knees, so your point of contact with the floor is your knees and palms. Push up off the floor while trying to keep your back straight. (This may be beyond the capacity of most of your participants, but it never hurts to try!)

Upper back strengthening

Lie face down on the floor, with your arms straight out to the sides from your shoulders. Lift your head, shoulders and arms off the floor, as if you were a giant bird flying. Keep your neck long.

Single leg lift for back-strengthening

In same starting position, lift one leg off the floor. Hold it for as long as you can, then lower. Try that with the other leg.

Buttock strengthening
As you lie face down on the floor, bend one leg up from the knee at right angles. Lift the bent leg off the floor. Now try this with the other leg.

Lying on the back on the floor

Knee hug stretch for hips, buttocks and lower back
Hug one knee up onto the chest, keeping the other leg stretched out on the floor. Repeat with the other leg.

Hip mobility
Keeping one leg flat on the floor, bend the other leg up to make a 90 degree angle. Let the raised leg drop slowly out to the floor sideways, hold it for a few seconds, then bring it slowly back in. Change over and repeat with the other leg.

Spinal release stretch
Lift your knees up to make right angles with the floor. Keep the knees slightly apart and in line with the hips, then gently rotate them to the right side and then the left.

Spinal rotation stretch
Lie with your legs stretched along the floor and your arms out wide to the side. Lift one knee up to your chest at a right angle, then allow it to drop over the opposite leg towards the floor at hip height. Bring to gently back to the centre, then change legs and try it on the other side.

Hamstring stretch lying
Bend one knee up onto the chest and rest your hand on the back of the thigh. Now try to straighten this leg. Support the leg by holding it with your hands.

Sit-ups for abdominal strengthening
Lie on your back, with knees bent up and your feet flat on the floor. Breathe in, then as you breathe out tuck your chin into chest and slowly lift your head and shoulders off the floor. Lift up your arms to help you balance. Can you see the other members of the class as you lift up? Hold this position for a minute, then breathe out as you come down slowly. How many times can you do this?

Oblique abdominal strengthening
Similar exercise as the one above, but as you come up, curl your body towards one knee. Repeat the exercise towards the other knee.

Quadriceps strengthening
Lie on your back, with one knee bent up and your foot placed flat on the floor. With the other leg held out straight, flex the foot and then lift it off the floor. Hold the leg in the air for a few counts, then slowly lower. Repeat with other leg.

> ## Safe dance tip: Coming up off the floor
>
> When coming up off the floor after an extended period, it is important to move slowly. The ideal way is to roll over onto the right side (away from the heart), and gradually bring the body to a sitting up position, then rest a few moments before standing. This reduces possible dizziness and low blood pressure from change in blood flow.

Standing exercises

These exercises are challenging for people with limited balance, so may only be appropriate with reasonably able groups.

Hamstring stretch standing
Place one foot out in front of you and pull your ankles and toes back towards you. Then lean your body forward over the outstretched leg and keep your back straight.

Combined hamstring and inner thigh stretch
Squat down with your knees open to the sides so that your hands are resting on the floor in front of you. Stretch out one leg to the side with the heel on the floor and the toes pulled back. If you want to stretch a bit harder, lean forward and keep your back straight.

Spine roll and release
To develop articulation of the spine and release of whole body after stretches. Place your feet about hip-width apart, with your arms relaxed by your sides and your knees relaxed. Allow your head to drop forward onto your chest and then towards the floor, followed gradually by the rest of the your body. Let your shoulders, upper back, middle back, then lower back (down as far as the coccyx) drop right forward. As your body drops, let your knees bend slightly. Let your whole body hang forward over your knees, arms and head relaxed and loose.

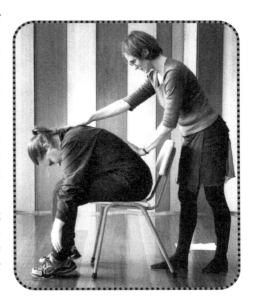

To return to standing position, begin by breathing in deeply and pulling in your stomach muscles. Slowly curl up by feeling each bone in your spine return to normal position. The last part of your body to come up should be your head.

Teaching tip: Developing articulation of the spine

The group leader stands behind the participant, firmly and carefully touching each vertebrae from the base of the skull down the spine to the coccyx. As each vertebrae is touched the participant releases that part of the back, allowing their torso and head to drop forward over their knees and their arms to hang heavily towards the floor. Then the group leader returns the participant to an upright position by touching each vertebrae from the coccyx up the spine. The head stays relaxed until the very last moment. Sometimes a gentle pull of the hair helps to position the head lightly and correctly on the top of the shoulders and to create a sense of release and lift through the whole body. This can also be done seated, as shown in this photo.

Shake-out to release muscular tension throughout the whole body

Give the whole body a good shake. Depending on how much time you have for this activity, you might just suggest a quick all-over shake or you could work through body parts in sections for greater focus and attention. Body part sections might be legs, feet, arms, hands, body, stomach, head, shoulders, all over. An excellent indepth reference on stretching is St George (1994), *The Stretching Handbook: 10 steps to muscle fitness.*

Music

Something flowing and mellow, but not too dreamy. The group leader needs to keep the energy of the group going here. Something like:

◎ The Cranberries, *No Need To Argue*

◎ Elvis Presley, *Love Songs.*

Theme: The body of the session

Usually this is the part of the session to which most time is allocated. Themes can range from exploring an imaginative concept through improvisation to learning the steps of a folk dance. You may find that some group members have very fertile imaginations and love to explore their ideas through dance. For example at BreakOut we have seen some people transform themselves into eagles, ducks and seagulls upon suggestion from the group leader. However, verbally communicating an imaginative concept will not always produce this result. There are some people who will only respond when they hear music and/or see movement happening around them. It is important for the group leader to recognise which approach suits each member and then find a way of bringing these approaches together so that each person can contribute to the session at their potential level.

Partner work

Listed below are some ideas that work well with a group of varying abilities. The aim of these is to develop focus and relationship, and extend both the range of movement and the experience of different qualities of movement. The activities also have a tactile element that can be an effective way of stimulating some people into movement. They also provide opportunities for group members to experience touch in a safe and sensitive manner.

There are many other possibilities for these kinds of activities. The more experienced you are as a leader, the more easily ideas for leading a session will come to you. You might use these as a starting point and find that your students lead you on to new ways of doing things.

Mirroring

Aims

Developing focus, eye contact, awareness of self and other, extending range of movement.

Props

White gloves can be effective in bringing the focus to the hands. A mask worn by one of the pair can be useful to clarify who the leader is. The mask can also help free up movement or create a

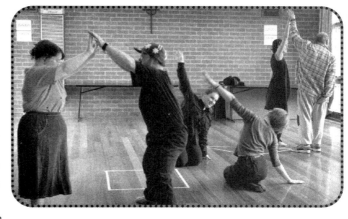

particular character or mood. This is then reflected back to the leader by the follower.

Description

Participants face a partner, about arm's length apart. To help people orient themselves and ensure that they are facing the right direction, ask them to look into their partner's eyes.

One person is the leader and the other is the follower. The leader's job is to improvise movements while the follower watches closely and mirrors those movements. The activity begins with the group leader demonstrating a movement as a starting point for the activity, for example, a circular movement of the hands and arms, like washing windows. The leader then builds on that movement to develop a sequence of his/her own, mirrored by the follower.

After a few minutes the leader brings his/her movement to an end and the roles are reversed. Music will help the flow of movement and can be used to give the cue to change roles.

Music

Something mellow and flowing:

- ◎ K.C. Wang (1996), *Chinese Bamboo Flute Songs*
- ◎ Cirque du Soleil (1998), *Collections*
- ◎ Enya (1997), *Paint the Sky with Stars*.

Follow the leader

Aims

Body contact, trust, attunement with partner.

Description

The *follower* stands behind the *leader* with their hands on the leader's shoulders. The *follower* closes his/her eyes and the *leader* carefully leads the *follower* around the room. After a few minutes the *leader* stops. Both pause for a moment and enjoy the stillness together, focusing on their breath while standing still. Then the *leader* walks around to stand behind his/her partner ready to be the *follower*. This can be done without music or with music that enhances the gentleness of the exercise.

Variation

The *follower* and the *leader* stay in their role. When the group leader gives the cue to stand still, the *leader* releases their hands from their partner's shoulders and moves to a new partner. The *follower* remains standing until a new partner becomes their *leader*. Repeat this three or four times and then swap over roles.

Music

Try this exercise without music first so that the *leader* can set his/her own pace, and the *follower* can really focus on the *leader*. Otherwise, something gentle and ambient such as:

- Tony O'Connor (1996), *Sea Australia*
- Pachelbel (1989), *Canon and Gigue and other Baroque Masterpieces*
- Daniel Scott (2000), *The Celtic Spirit*, also available with accompanying book of poems: Scott (2000), *The Celtic Spirit: Poems, Prayers and Music*.

Pushing/pulling/melting

Aims

Body contact, trust, developing strength and control, moving and lengthening the body vertically and horizontally.

Description

- *Brick wall pushing:* Partners stand facing each other about 1 metre apart, feet firmly on the ground. The two make contact by pressing their palms together, then increasing pressure so that they are pushing with all their strength. The group leader could suggest imagining that the partner is a brick wall they want to push down.

- *Back to back pushing:* This exercise can also be done standing back to back.

- *Pushing up and down from the floor:* This exercise focuses on moving in the vertical plane. Pushing can be used to achieve standing and sitting, but will require a lot of physical strength and co-operation between partners. A staff member should be on hand to offer support when needed as this is a challenging exercise for those with low muscle tone.

  Partners sit back to back on the floor with their elbows interlocked, knees bent up and feet placed firmly on the ground close to their buttocks. Both partners push into each other's back, using all their strength to push together and then push up. This will create the impetus to move from sitting to standing. Once standing, participants push again into their partner's back and bend their knees slowly. As their knees bend, the weight of their bodies will draw them back down to the ground.

- *Pulling and reaching:* This exercise focuses on moving in the horizontal plane. Partners hold each other's hands as if they were shaking hands. Then they stretch out their arms to make one long line between the two bodies. The group leader can encourage participants to stretch with their free hand to the nearest window or door and imagine that their arms are made of elastic or chewing gum. The aim is to gradually lengthen the arms and the distance between partners and then hold the tension. Once this point of tension is achieved, participants can let go of their partner's hand and continue to reach towards the wall or window with their free hand. This can be a sustained release like a piece of chewing gum separating or a sudden release like a 'snap' when something breaks.

The exercise can continue with participants reaching out to find a new partner and starting again. Or, like a stretched elastic band being released, partners can snap back towards each other and finish standing shoulder to shoulder.

◎ *Melting:* Partners stand back to back feeling relaxed. The group leader brings awareness to specific body parts by saying in a soft voice, 'Relax shoulders, back, pelvis, knees, etc…..'. Participants should be given time to become aware of each body part. The group leader can also bring awareness to the contact that is being made between the two bodies. She/he could say to the group, 'Can you feel your partner's shoulders?' Once this awareness is established, partners rock gently together from side to side. Water imagery can help the body relax. The group might imagine they are on a boat being rocked gently by the water. This activity can also be done sitting back to back on the floor.

Music
Gentle music without strong beat, but not too dreamy, for example, nature sounds like Track 2, Tribal Trance (1988), *Minjarah*, or a subdued classical piece like Café del Mar (1999) *Arias 2: New Horizon.*

Sounds can be used to accompany movement. For example, as participants pull away from their partners in the reaching exercise, they could try making a long whistle or an 'ooooooo' sound. Experimentation with sounds during the warm-up will help people become familiar with the concept when it comes to putting sound and movement together. This will also give participants ideas of sounds they can make. Vowel sounds are always a good place to start.

Sculptor and clay

Aims
Touch requiring sensitivity and respect, body part and shape awareness, co-operation, experiencing and observing movement, leadership.

Description
Working in pairs, one person is the *clay* and the other the *sculptor*. The *clay* is the person who is moved and the *sculptor* is the person who makes the *clay* move. The *clay* stands in a neutral position (relaxed) and the *sculptor* chooses a part of the *clay's* body to move. For example, the *clay's* hand is moved and placed on his/her own shoulder. One body part is moved at a time, for example, after the hand the head is moved so that the clay is looking over their right shoulder. The *sculptor* continues to move the *clay* until she/he is happy with the position created. The *sculptor* then stands back and looks closely at the shape of their partner's body and walks around their creation to admire it from different angles.
Sculptor and *clay* swap over roles.

Initially the group leader may need to direct the activity by specifying to the *sculptor* which body parts to move. When participants become familiar with the exercise and are at ease with their partner, the group leader can decrease their leadership and encourage the *sculptor* to make decisions independently.

Music

This is a good exercise to do without music to reduce limits on the decisions of the *sculptor*. When participants become confident in their decision-making, music can add another dimension. See what the difference is if the background music is sharp and when it is flowing. Are the shapes different? Also try different soundscapes like the sea, bush, rainforest.

- ◉ Sharp Music: Balanesque Quartet, *Possessed*
- ◉ Flowing Music: *Great Dream Classics*
- ◉ Soundscapes: Tony O'Connor, *Sea Australia*.

Group sculpture

Aims

Using the whole body to form shapes, forming shapes in relationship to one or more people, individual decision-making, group co-operation.

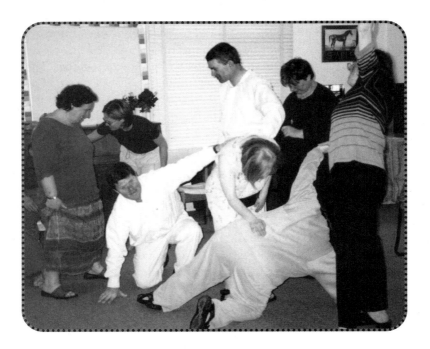

Description

The group leader designates an area in the dance space as the sculpture building site, perhaps the centre of the room. One person initiates the process by forming a shape in this spot and holding it still. The next person enters the space and finds a point of connection with the person holding their shape. For example, the person entering extends their hand so that the palm of their hand is touching the outstretched palm of the person holding the shape. One by one, group members enter to build the shape.

Variations

◎ *Small groups:* If the group is large you could build a number of small sculptures in groups of three. Begin by having the whole group arrange themselves in a large circle around the designated 'building site', so that everyone can watch the emerging shapes. Groups can be pre-set if this level of facilitation is needed, or group members can respond spontaneously to the shape emerging. Once the third person has joined the sculpture, the group leader can indicate the end of the activity by saying 'thank you' or 'freeze'. This can be a signal to release the shape and move back to the circle.

◎ *Set a theme:* The group can decide on a theme, so that there is an intention behind the shapes made by each person. Some examples are a flock of birds, people at a picnic, a city skyline.

◎ *Changing shape:* This can be done with small or large groups. Once the last person has entered and formed their shape, participants all take a deep breath, and on the out breath, release the shape and carefully shift into another position. The aim is to make subtle shifts in shape instead of an entirely new position.

◎ *Moving sculptures*: Instead of the first person forming a shape and holding it, they choose a spot on the site and create a simple repetitive movement such as standing still and swinging arms in opposition. One by one, group members enter the space, placing themselves in relationship to the person or people already there, for example, kneeling or sitting next to someone. Each person follows the same repetitive movement or a variation of it. It can be fun to add sounds to the movement such as 'swish', 'oosh', 'ooo'. The movement itself may inspire a spontaneous sound response, or the leader can ask for suggestions.

Music

All these exercises can be done effectively without music. Music, however, can help relax the group, support a theme or inspire ideas. If the group is aiming to create a static sculpture, avoid music with a strong beat.

◎ Background music: Café del Mar *Aria 2*.

◎ Theme music: 'Sea Australia' (gentle seascape music), *Possessed,* The Balanescu Quartet (excellent for industrial sounds).

Further reading

◎ Helen Payne's (1994) book, *Creative Movement and Dance in Group Work* has many more ideas for activities.

Improvisation and solos

At BreakOut, we often schedule time for group members to create their own movements. This provides opportunities for participants to develop their own style, as well as confidence to perform for an audience. Ideas that come from improvisation often inspire the group in new ways.

Improvised performances

Aims

Development of creativity, confidence, performance skills, observation skills, decision making, personal style and opportunity for choice.

Description

Firstly the performance space should be defined. There are two options:

- The group makes a large circle and the performer uses the space in the middle. This way the group remains close to the performer and the performer is supported by the power of the circle.

- A more traditional performance space is set up with the audience sitting at the front and the performer using the space like a stage. With this arrangement there is a separation between the performer and the group, making the performer more exposed and more vulnerable. These feelings may need to be explored by the individual and the group with the help of the group leader.

There are different ways to proceed from here. The following are some ideas:

Participants choose their own music

The group leader can display a selection of CDs from which a choice can be made. Some people may like to bring their own music to increase the variety experienced by the group. Different music will create different ways of moving. For example, music with a strong beat can encourage stamping and jumping, while soft flowing music usually encourages swaying of arms and body. A person can be drawn to explore movements beyond their preferred style through the use of music with different qualities. The key is to offer lots of choice and to encourage participants to try something new.

The group leader makes the choice of music to help extend movement range

For example, there may be a predominance of light or weightless movement in the group. This way of moving is often seen in people with autism, especially those who walk on their toes. Dance can provide the experience of moving so that weight moves down through the body to the feet, with movements like marching, stomping and jumping. Music with a strong beat, such as African drumming music, can be very effective in bringing weight into movement.

When there is a predominance of strong, weighted movement in the group, which can often be the case with people with cerebral palsy who have high body tone and bound flow movement, the leader can try some light classical music. This may inspire a flow of movement through the torso and arms. A good selection of classical music can be found in ABC Classics (1998), *The Swoon Collections*.

Set a theme

◎ Nature is a good source for imaginative ideas, as most people have an experience of the natural environment from which to draw on. For example, following the journey of a river. This activity could begin with a discussion about rivers. Participants can discover words to describe the movement of a river such as fast, still, slow, tumbling. Then explore those ideas through movement.

◎ A scene from everyday life, such as getting up in the morning, can also be a good starting point. Yawning and stretching could be explored as an activity. Participants could begin by stretching just one part of the body at a time, such as one arm, before stretching out the whole body. The exercise could continue with exploration of the relationship between extension and contraction. For example, members might imagine stretching out their bodies, then drawing back into a snug position as if in bed. It can be fun to add the sounds of yawning to the movement.

◎ *Some other thematic ideas:* Taking a train journey, trying on some new clothes, walking along the beach, being in the middle of a big storm, travelling into outer space, having a bad hair day, meeting a new friend, kicking through autumn leaves.

Using props

Display a variety of props from which group members can choose. Some suggestions include balloons, scarves, fans, masks, cloaks, shawls, big boots, tambourines, drums, castanets, swords and shields. A prop may be enough to excite participants' imaginations, though the group leader may need to be prepared to lead participants through an exploration of what the prop can do or what it can suggest. This activity can begin with participants simply touching, holding or trying on the props, then being encouraged to find out what they can do with the prop. The exploration of props may suggest movements such as waving a fan, swaying with a shawl or beating a drum.

To extend imaginative thinking, the group leader might then ask members to describe the prop: 'Tell us what your big boots look like?' She/he might ask participants to define the feeling they get when using the prop: 'How do you feel when you are wearing your big boots?', and then demonstrate the movement qualities inspired by the prop: 'Can you show me how you move in your big boots?' A final step might be to ask participants to describe the movement in words: 'What kind of movements did you make when you were wearing your boots?'

A character, mood or place may emerge out of this discussion that could inspire further exploration through improvisation or even the choreography of a dance piece. For example, the big boots could be space boots. From this idea the group might experiment using big floaty steps as if moonwalking, then improvise around the theme of being weightless in space.

For more ideas about props, see Chapter 5.

Music

◎ Tribal Trance (1998), *Minjahra.* Excellent selection of music from flowing to strong rhythms.

◎ Mickey Hart (1991), *Planet Drum*, great drumming music and vocals

◎ Jan Garbeck & The Hilliard Ensemble (1994), *Officium*, gentle and haunting

◎ Bert Kaempfert, *Roses,* tracks 10–14, playful.

Exploring dynamics of movement

As described earlier in this chapter, all movement can be described in terms of Laban's Effort Dynamics: Weight, Space, Flow and Time, (defined by the polarities of strength and lightness, direct and indirect spatial intentions, bound and free flow, suddenness and sustainment). Movement travels in different directions (forwards, backwards, sideways and diagonally) and occurs on a range of levels (high, low and medium). Many interesting movement and dance experiences can be explored simply by playing with these dynamics.

> ### Teaching tip: Finding your own space
>
> An important concept in a room full of moving people is the idea of one's own space; that is, a place where one can stand on a spot and move without touching another person or object. A double armspan is an ideal distance for one's own space, i.e. both arms should be able to stretch out wide and swing around without restriction.

Moving with variation in time, level and weight

Aims

Extending movement experience beyond personal preference, experiencing contrast in movement, spatial awareness, responding to change.

Description

Time (suddenness/sustainment)

Taking control: Participants walk at their normal pace without stopping. When the group leader calls out 'freeze', everyone stops. 'Go' is the cue for movement to continue. The length of time between each 'freeze' can be lengthened or shortened so that it comes as a surprise. Participants will need to remain alert and in control of their movement to be ready to stop at any moment.

It may be difficult for some people with physical disabilities, low stamina or poor concentration to engage in or sustain movement. Participants with physical disabilities will need a moderate to slow pace, with carefully prompted dynamic changes, while those with poor concentration are likely to be more engaged if dynamic changes are short and sharp. For participants with an abundance of flow in their bodies, like some people with Down syndrome, it is difficult to have the control to stop. A strong cue such as a gong or drum beat can help bring alertness into the body and make stopping easier.

Variation

The class can be divided into two. One group dashes (suddenness), while the other glides (sustainment). This activity could begin with one group frozen in position, and then develop so that both groups are moving simultaneously.

Levels (high/medium/low)

Participants find their own space in the room. The leader directs the group to relax all parts of the body, then imagine they are like icecreams melting on a hot day or candles slowly burning down. Once they have melted down to the floor, the group can then explore moving at a low level on backs or stomachs, using arms and legs to push the body along the floor. Then participants stop all movement and lie still for a moment. Next, they imagine that a piece of string is attached to one hand like a puppet string. This pulls the person up slowly from the floor, perhaps into a full stretch with arms reaching towards the ceiling and spine lengthening. Finally, participants imagine that the string is cut and their arms fall down. They finish by standing relaxed. Once participants are experienced at coming up off the floor with movement initiated in the arms, they could experiment with possibilities like attaching strings to more than one body part, or to different parts (feet, head, chest, etc.). See what happens when you try and come off the floor chest first!

Weight (lightness, strength and heaviness)

Participants walk around the room, imagining they are walking on clouds, making their steps as light as possible so they don't fall through (lightness). When everyone is moving lightly, the image changes and the cloud becomes a cardboard box. The group stamps and stomps until the box is a flat piece of board on the ground (strength). The image changes again and the cardboard becomes a delicate piece of cloth that will float away unless weighed down by something heavy. Bodies sink into the floor so that their weight holds the cloth down (heaviness).

Music

◎ **Lightness:** Mozart (1998) *Clarinet Concerto in A Major,
The Great Dream Classics* (1998)

◎ **Strength:** Orff, *Carmina Burana*

◎ **Heaviness:** Bach (1998), 'Air on a G String', *The Great Dream Classics* (1998).

Group members could also make their own music with rhythm sticks. These can be made simply out of sticks of wood or purchased at a music shop. One group could make the sound while the other moves.

Variations

◎ *Develop a sequence.* This is best if done in small groups of three to four people. Each person chooses one dynamic and these are put together in a sequence. For example, the sequence could be moving lightly, moving backwards slowly, moving forwards fast, sinking to the floor and then starting at the beginning again. The group could create their own sounds to accompany the sequence or fit it to a piece of someone's favourite music.

◎ *Sharing leadership.* Participants take it in turns to choose a dynamic with which to lead the group.

◎ *Create a character:* Depending upon the nature of the group, it may be possible to develop these exercises into imaginative play. Members can discuss what they are thinking or feeling while they are moving and perhaps define a situation or character that encapsulates these. Through movement improvisation, the character or situation could take on a life of its own, giving expression to the imaginative and feeling life of the person.

Group improvisation: From the moon to the jungle

In one session, we all began by moving around the room with light steps, imagining we were walking on the moon. Arms began to float in the air and steps became bigger and lighter. Then I (Jenny) jumped and made a big thud and began to walk with strong heavy steps. As I looked around I saw that other people's arms had begun swinging and feet were hitting the ground. Group member John saw the opportunity to transform into an elephant and began swinging his arms like a trunk. Very quickly there was a room full of elephants and one monkey. Valerie always looks for the opportunity to do something different to the rest of the group and this time her monkey was a creative expression of rebellion. She was having so much fun that she successfully recruited some of the elephants to be monkeys. We could no longer hear the background music as the chuckles of the monkeys and the roar of the elephants filled the room. We finished by collapsing on the floor and having a good laugh.

I asked John what he had been thinking about while he was moving. He replied with a big roar, 'An elephant of course'. He then said he was strong and lived in a jungle. I asked him whether he liked feeling strong and he stood up, banged on his chest like Tarzan and said, 'Of course I do'.

Through experimenting with his weight in movement, John was able to explore the feeling of being a big strong animal. He was also able to tell the group that he liked feeling strong. This was a reminder to me that people who are often unable to speak or advocate for themselves still have a desire to be heard, respected and valued.

Relaxation

Relaxation activities can be used ritualistically as part of the closure of sessions. These can also be useful to help participants regain focus or reduce agitation or fatigue during the session. All of these activities take some getting used to. Participants may at first resist new experiences, but in time generally come to enjoy the contact. One carer told us that she particularly requested being on duty on Saturday mornings so that she could enjoy shoulder massages at BreakOut with her client. Ideally all staff should experience these activities themselves before they do them to others, so they can imagine how a participant feels as their body is being manipulated.

These activities require different levels of energy from staff. Sometimes the group leader and assistants, as well as participants, might be exhausted at the end of a session, and need an activity that is not too demanding. On other days it might be possible to offer an activity that requires a more intense level of input, particularly if there is a high staff to participant ratio. The following activities have been ordered in terms of energy level, to help the group leader select what might be appropriate in their circumstances.

Teaching tip: Constructive rest pose

The safest position for lying on the floor is constructive rest pose, i.e. with the back flat on the floor, knees together, bent up at a 90 degree angle with feet flat on the floor about 60 cm apart and the hands and arms flat on the floor. This position reduces pressure on the spine and neck and allows the back to flatten out comfortably.

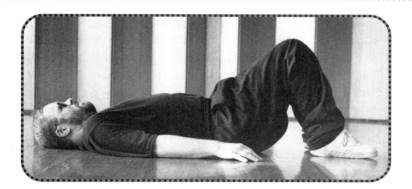

Guided imagery

Aims

This activity can be relaxing for everyone. It's a good one for a day when things haven't gone so well and staff are out of energy. It is most suitable for class members with reasonable capacity to understand verbal language without visual cues.

Description

Participants sit or lie in a comfortable position (ideally constructive rest pose), with their eyes closed. If they are on chairs, their spines should be well-supported, arms and hands relaxed by the sides of their bodies or in their laps, with their chests open and shoulders relaxed. Heads might be dropped forward onto chests, with eyes closed.

Using a low steady voice, the leader can talk the group through an imagined scene. This might be:
- a sunbake on a warm beach
- a float in fluffy clouds
- a meander through a Balinese water garden
- a stroll in a rainforest.

The description should be multisensory; including descriptions of what participants might see, hear, smell, touch and feel. Appropriate music can really help set the scene.

Music
- Howling Wind (1995), *Dugong Lullaby,* atmospheric tracks for sea/forest outdoor themes
- Enya (1997), *Paint the Sky with Stars*, Tracks 12, 13, 15 suitable for floating scenes
- Steve Parrish, Les Gilbert (1996), *Cry of the River Forest*, Australian nature sounds-ideal for imagery of birds and nature.

Seated stretch with scarves

Aims
Suitable cool-down activity for participants who prefer to be seated in chairs.

Description
Class members stretch out, using scarves held in both hands. Scarves for this activity need to be long and narrow. They should not be too slippery so participants can get a good grip. Satin scarves can be frustratingly elusive when one tries to position them underfoot.

- *Body and back stretch:* Hold the scarf up high, and stretch out your arms as wide as you can. Now take a deep breath in and bend to the right and feel your whole body stretching. Come back to the middle and try it to the other side.

   Can you reach forward with your scarf – perhaps touching scarves with someone across the circle? Then let your head drop forward and let your scarf drop right down to the floor. Let your head hang heavy over your knees.

   While you are down there – can you take your scarf in one hand and swish it on the ground around your feet? Can you reach beside the chair? Behind the chair? In front of the chair? Now try it with the other arm and hand.

   Taking a deep slow breath in – come slowly to a sitting up position.

- *Arm stretch:* Using only one hand this time, can you make your scarf fly up and down? Let your arm flick so that your scarf really flies. Imagine the wind is blowing through your scarf so that it makes patterns in the air. Can you move it sideways as well? Try it with the other arm too.

- *Body twist:* This time, twist your body around as if you want to dust cobwebs away from the air. Can you dust right out in front of you – to the side, behind you? Imagine there are lots of cobwebs behind you. See if you can get rid of them all. Can you try it on the other side also?

- *Leg and feet stretch:* Now it is time to stretch out your legs and feet. Can you loop the scarf under one foot? Pull on the scarf to lift and straighten out your leg. Can you pull your toes towards you and feel a stretch right down the back of your leg? How high can you lift your leg? Do it with the other leg as well.

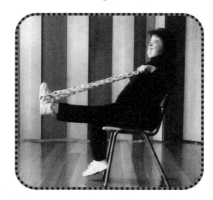

Could you try lifting both legs at once? Hold on tight to your scarf for balance, or even the back of your chair.

◎ *Neck and head stretch:* The last parts of the body to stretch out are your head and neck. Can you put the scarf around behind your head and gently pull on it so that your head comes forward on to your chest?

Let go of your scarf and continue stretching. Let your head drop to the right side, imagining that your ear is falling towards your shoulder. Try this to the left side as well. Then gently turn your head to look at the person on your right. Can you look at the person on your left as well?

◎ *Relaxation:* Finish this activity by letting go of your scarf and letting it drop down to the floor. Imagine yourself as relaxed and still as that scarf on the floor. Let your breath come in and out slowly a few times. You might like to close your eyes so you can just think about breathing, in and out, in and out.

◎ *Wake up and shake-out:* Now slowly open your eyes and have a look around the circle to bring yourself back to the group. Smile at anyone you see. Give yourself a little shake all over to get your blood moving again; feet, legs, arms, hands, chest, stomach, head.

Music

◎ Marisa Robles (1992), *The World of the Harp*, Track 5, ideal for a 'slowing down', but not a 'stopping' activity.

◎ J.S. Bach/ The Academy of Ancient Music (1997), *Solo and Double Violin Concertos*.

Relaxation with props

Aims

Using a prop can add interest and is sometimes useful for helping class members reach an altered state of consciousness through relaxation.

Description

Flying Wave: This activity involves the manipulation of a giant piece of fabric in waves above participants' heads. We have often used this one in classes for children, but began using it with adults too when one day I had the opportunity to be on the floor underneath it, and enjoyed the sense of magic and peace it created. The nicest wave we have is a silky stretch fabric, deep blue colour flecked with small silver stars. In combination with the gentle starry music, it really has a very relaxing effect on those underneath it.

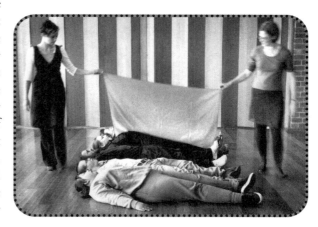

Participants lie on their backs on the floor in a long row. The group leader and assistant each take one end of a long piece of soft fabric (approx. 1 x 2 metres) and gently walk up and down the length of the room, allowing the fabric to float over the bodies of those lying down, not touching, but close enough for the movement of air to be felt. The floating fabric can also be directed specifically at one person, with the leader and assistant standing at the head and feet of person and floating the fabric up and then right down over and onto their body. This is a lovely way to help a person get a sense of their whole body, the connectedness of it. It is an activity that is particularly useful for those with sensory integration difficulties, or those with poor body concept and co-ordination.

Music
◎ Enya (1997), *Paint the Sky with Stars*
◎ or 'Under African Skies', *Out of Africa* soundtrack.

Variation
Spine roller: A spine roller is a handheld wooden gadget with two small moving wheels. Participants lie face down on the floor, with their arms stretched out to the side. The group leader uses the spine roller to give the participant an all-over massage, up and down the spine, across the shoulders, along the arms, down the legs. Firm, slow pressure is ideal, to allow participants the chance to really engage in the experience of body parts being 'rolled'.

Shaving brush massage: A shaving brush can be used to give a massage to participants who prefer to stay seated. Heads, shoulders, face, necks and hands can be lightly brushed with a shaving brush for a very relaxing experience.

> ## Teaching tip: Issues about intimate physical contact
> Sometimes it is advisable to reduce or eliminate close physical contact between a group leader and a participant. For example, between people who don't know each other well, between cross-gender partners, i.e. female group leader and a male participant where there may be issues of appropriateness of intimate physical contact, for participants who are sensitive to touch like some people with autism or those who are very ticklish, or those who are having issues to do with managing their sexuality. A relaxation activity like the spine roller activity above is ideal, as it affords the participant a sense of massage and awareness of body parts, without involving actual physical contact.

Head, neck and shoulder massage
◎ *Shoulders, neck and back:* Stand behind the participant. Begin by working the muscles in and around their neck and shoulders with firm squeezing movements. The area of muscles where the shoulders and head join can become very tense. Move across the top of the shoulders, over the shoulder blades, then down the back, rubbing the muscular areas with firm, slow pressure. It can be helpful to tip the person forward over their knees to give better access to the back and spine, while also stretching out the muscles of the back. Gradually knead your way back to the top of the spine, then across the shoulders to the top of one arm. Knead your way down that arm with firm pressure. Take the palm of the hand between your own, and flatten and lengthen fingers with a sharp downward pull. Make your way up and across to the other arm and repeat on the other side.

◉ *Head massage:* The final part of the body massage is for the head and scalp. Begin by taking large clumps of the person's hair and gently pull them away from their scalp. This sounds gruesome, but is actually a very relaxing and freeing experience if it is done with exactly the right pressure. Do this over the whole scalp. Complement this hair-raising experience with firm slow handstrokes over the whole scalp, as if you were smoothing out a mussed hairstyle.

◉ *Head press:* Place the palm of one of your hands firmly against the participant's forehead and the other on the back of their neck near the base of the skull. Apply firm even pressure for several minutes to both front and back of the skull, then release gradually.

◉ *Earlobe stretch:* The final part of the relaxation: take hold of one earlobe in each hand and pull down very gently. After a minute or so, gradually ease off the pressure and let your hands slowly float up into the air. This will move the participant's energy on and upward, appropriate for the transition to another activity.

Teaching tip

When massaging use firm, slow pressure. This reduces sensations of tickling and helps the participant get a stronger sense of the body part being worked on. Try to keep physical contact with the participant at all times so they can anticipate the next body part to be touched. If you need to change sides, or walk around their chair, keep one hand or finger in actual contact with them, so they know where you are. Fewer surprises means more trust and a deeper level of relaxation that can be reached.

Spine stretch

Aims

To assist group members to develop a greater sense of their spine and its articulation (feeling each vertebrae separately).

Description

Spine outline: Start with fingers on the top of the neck, touching the atlas, (first cervical vertebra below the skull). Then using the fingers of both hands, with firm pressure trace down each vertebra of the spine. Encourage the participant to allow their body to relax and fall forward, as if you were releasing each vertebra as you touched it. By the time you reach the coccyx (the base bone of the spine, between the top of the buttocks), the participant's body should be dropped right forward with their chest over their thighs. Allow them to relax there for a minute, then reach forward to slowly lift their hands and arms up and over their head, thereby bringing their torso up too. Stretch their arms behind their head a little, giving their spine an opposite stretch to the forward C-curve they have just made over their knees. Stand close behind them for this activity, with your body weight against their back. This will help support their head, neck and spine as you stretch

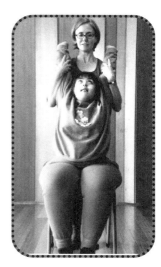

them backwards. Encourage them to release their shoulders and open their chest as they go backwards. Lastly, slowly bring their arms down to rest in their lap, and bring their spine back to vertical.

Full body stretch

Aims
Class members lie on the floor on their backs, arms relaxed by their sides. Group leader and assistants travel around the room visiting each member in turn to give them a full body stretch.

Description
Legs: The leader is positioned squatting or kneeling on the floor facing participant's feet. He or she takes hold of the participant's legs at the back of the ankle and gently pulls their legs away from their body, lengthening legs parallel with the floor and torso of participant.

Arms and spine: the leader is positioned squatting behind the participant's head. He or she reaches forward to take hold of participant's arms, gently pulling them up and over the head, away from the shoulders, flattening out palms and fingers back down on to the floor. This activity lengthens arms, releases shoulder joints and lengthens upper spine.

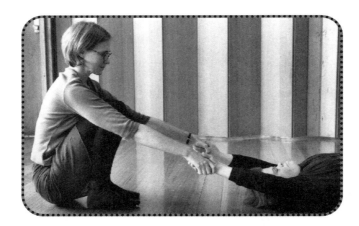

Head: Still positioned behind the participant's head, the group leader gently puts both hands under the participant's neck, cradling their head. Very gently, the head is pulled away from the shoulders, releasing and lengthening the neck before being gently laid down again on the floor.

This activity often takes quite a while to feel comfortable with. The participant needs to be encouraged to trust the leader and give over control of their body, to relax and feel heavy. After this stretch, the body feels really long and released, as if there were a lot of space between the bones, reversing the compressing effects of gravity and age.

Closure

A ritual closure is the ideal way to mark the end of a session. Clients, carers and families will all be clear when the session has finished if you do this. After the relaxation period, when class members have separated into their own private space, it can be satisfying to reconnect energy.

Group hug

Aims
Expression of friendship, enjoyable physical contact, group connectedness.

Description
Each group member in the circle reaches out to the people on either side of them and gives them a hug.

Well done!

Aims
Encourages physical contact and vocal expression – especially good for those with autism, enjoyable for all.

Description
The whole class is positioned in a circle, in close body contact. Each member reaches out to the people on either side and pats them both on the back, congratulating each other physically and verbally for effort and achievement in the session.

Group bow, stretch and clap

Aims
This activity clearly marks the end of the session and in doing so creates a transition from the dance session to the outside world.

Description
The whole class is positioned in a circle holding hands. Hands are raised above the head and held until everyone has found this position. Then all arms come down and participants simultaneously bend at the waist. Arms keep moving until the hands touch the ground or get as close as possible. Knees should soften as members bend and reach. Hands lift over the head once again, then release from holding and drop by the side. The last movement can be accompanied by a big breath and vocalising 'aaah' (like a sigh) as the hands drop down. Standing upright altogether, the group gives themselves a big clap.

Variations
⊚ *Individually*: same as above without holding hands
⊚ *Mexican Wave Style:* Stand in a circle and begin the above activity with one person. The gesture then moves around the circle. The designated starter lifts arms above their head and then drops them down to their side. The next person begins to lift their arms when they see the person before them begin to lower their arms. The gesture continues around the circle until it reaches the beginning again. This can be repeated several times with increase and decrease in speed.
⊚ *Stomping:* Try stomping instead of clapping for the finale.

Chapter 3

Working with children who have special needs

Creative dance classes provide the opportunity for children with special needs to engage in play, movement and the world of imagination in a social context. For many reasons, including the amount of time needed to care for the child's basic needs, this may not naturally happen within the child's home environment. Creative dance can be beneficial for a child's development in every aspect: physical, cognitive, language, social and emotional.

A children's group leader needs to have energy, enthusiasm and patience. While the processes are similar to those used with adult groups, more physical energy is required when working with children. As a facilitator, it is important to fully enter the world of the child in movement and imagination, and to enjoy sharing this experience with them.

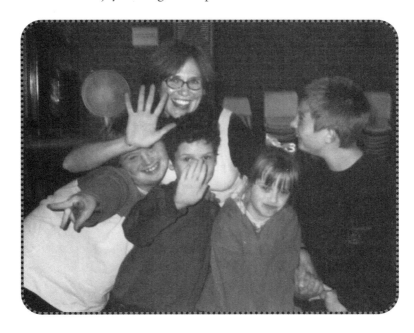

In Chapter 7 we will look at strategies for successfully running a group dance session in detail. Most of these strategies also apply when working with children. Some additional concepts are described below.

Managing the group

Use the child's name

Use the child's name first whenever you speak to them. Children may need to hear their own name, even when comments are being made to the whole group to ensure that focus is maintained.

Keep the dance space relatively quiet and orderly, at least until children are comfortable and have mastered the basic techniques.

Rules for the dance space

Begin the dance program by establishing basic rules, such as:

- keep talking to a minimum. In the dance session, we are communicating with our bodies and our movements
- when one person is talking, everyone else listens
- work in your own space unless asked by the teacher to work with someone else (this is a positive way to say no touching.)
- respect everyone's ideas and efforts. In this program, there is no right or wrong way.

Finding your own space

Children may need to be introduced to the concept of one's own space. This can be done initially by placing a marker on the floor for each child to stand on, such as a cross of masking tape. Another way to define one's own space is to ask children to extend their arms as wide as they can and to move away from anyone they are touching.

Keep language positive

As far as possible, use positive language to give feedback to children. Notice group members who are participating co-operatively rather than those who are not. Comment on the things you see that you like, that are interesting, that are unusual. If you notice only positive and co-operative behaviours, those children who want to draw attention to themselves by misbehaving will soon figure out that the best way to get your attention is to try their hardest to do what you have asked. Dance may be a time when children who do not get positive feedback in other learning contexts can be rewarded by acknowledgment.

Managing disruptions

For children who are having trouble managing themselves, the strategic use of a quiet spot in the room may help. Children can rejoin the group when they are ready to follow the rules (the teacher, aide or child can decide when is the right time to rejoin the group).

Staffing issues: Ratio of staff to students

A group leader running a dance program for children with special needs should have appropriate support. A good ratio is one adult to four children. This may vary depending on the support needs and level of ability of the children.

Clarify roles of staff

A group leader working with assistants, aides or classroom teachers, should clarify roles for all staff before the program begins. One approach I (Kim) have used when working as a visiting specialist with classroom teachers is to deal with the content of the session, paying attention to those who are participating well. I have left issues of misbehaviour and discipline to the classroom teacher. Children who want my attention need to co-operate. Classroom teachers and aides can be encouraged to join in with dance activities as they feel comfortable. Children often really enjoy seeing their classroom teachers face a challenge or a new activity with them.

Leading the session

Ensure clarity of session structure

Create a clear beginning, middle and end to each session with distinct cues that mark the transition from one section to another. For example, sitting in a circle could indicate the beginning of the session, standing could be the beginning point for the active middle section and lying on the floor could be the cue for the quieter relaxation section at the end. These very distinct movement cues are helpful in uniting the group at the different stages of transition.

Simplicity is the best starting place

It is a good strategy to develop movement experiences from a simple concept. The following example shows how a simple idea can be extended into a more complex exercise. You can think about this in terms of adding layers of complexity.

- ◉   An initial activity might be moving and stopping.
- ◉   Next stage: moving and stopping with a partner.
- ◉   Next stage: moving, stopping with partner, and when stopped connecting both hands with the partner's to make an archway.
- ◉   Next stage: moving, stopping with partner, and when stopped making a different shape with partner using hands and arms.

Depending on the group, this might be achievable in one or two sessions. A good way to introduce new ideas is to repeat the basic exercise every week, gradually adding another stage at each new session. This approach gives time for new concepts to be integrated into the body.

Age-appropriate music

Children are generally very responsive to music that has a happy feel and a lot of 'bounce'. They will enjoy dancing to songs from their favourite TV show or film, and can be encouraged to bring their favourite music to class. Music that is used to inspire movement needs to be very clear. Select tapes or CDs that have simple melodies and rhythms, with not too many instruments playing at the same time. Give the children plenty of opportunities to listen to a wide variety of music. Music from the classical western tradition and folk traditions (world music) will encourage interesting possibilities for expressing ideas, emotions and movement.

Props and sensory stimulation

Use props with different textures, colours and sounds to stimulate touch, hearing and sight. Props will also engage the imagination and help some children participate more fully in the dance session, especially those with autism who relate more easily to objects than people. Chapter 5 includes many more ideas about props.

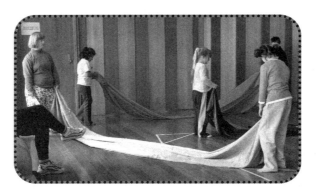

Additional theoretical concepts

Developmental movement principles

In addition to Laban's theories discussed in Chapter 2, the developmental movement principles of Body–Mind Centering are useful when working with children. These are 'based on the natural development and unfolding of potential within the human being' (Hartley, 1995) and were developed by American dancer, occupational therapist and movement educator Bonnie Bainbridge Cohen.

These principles acknowledge that:

⊚ there are differences in the timing and progress of each child's physical skills and co-ordination and that this needs to be taken into account when planning a dance program

⊚ human movement development occurs in a layered fashion. Early movement patterns such as sitting, rolling, creeping, crawling, etc. underlie and support the emergence of more sophisticated movement patterns, such as walking, running, jumping, skipping and turning. To assist children to master more complex movement skills, we return to earlier movement patterns to support their development.

⊚ Yielding, pushing, reaching and pulling are four fundamental experiences in movement development.
  • Yielding involves learning how to rest actively and relate to a surface such as the floor (earth), or another person (being held or cuddled).
  • Pushing involves pushing with the head or tail through the spine, pushing with the feet/legs or hands/arms.
  • Reaching involves moving beyond one's personal space by extending a part of the body, for example, reaching out to grab something.
  • Pulling involves gathering or taking hold of something and bringing it towards oneself (Wishart, 2000).

The 3 Rs of movement – rhythm, repetition and ritual

David Wells, improvisation artist and teacher, refers to these very effective practices – rhythm, ritual and repetition, for working with children (Wishart, 2000).

◉ Rhythm can be established in a group by clapping, stomping or making body percussion. A group rhythm brings focus and connectedness to a group that is an important dynamic for the start of a session. Establishing rhythm can be as simple as singing a 'hello song' accompanied by clapping. This can be very alluring to the child who has withdrawn from the group as they can experience the enjoyment and energy that is building up within the group from the outside.

◉ Repetition involves doing a movement experience over and over again so that the body is given time to integrate the pattern. New skills can be mastered through repetition, and children love to repeat movements they enjoy.

◉ Ritual involves establishing a routine that becomes well known to children. The familiarity of regular activities assists the establishment of trust, stability and identity of a group. The anticipation of well-loved rituals can bring about a joyful excitement in participants.

Working with special needs children in integrated settings (school classrooms, dance studios, recreational programs, after-school care)

Children with mild disabilities or special needs may benefit the most from participating in a mainstream dance program. The challenge for a group leader of such a program is to ensure that the child's special needs are met, while also accommodating the abilities of others in the group. The Laban methodology is ideal in this situation as it actively encourages and values difference and does not require mastery of any particular body skills to achieve educational goals. This distinguishes the Laban approach from other styles of dance that are popular with children, such as jazz or classical ballet. These dance styles are more likely to magnify the differences and limitations of children with special needs because of their prescriptive movement vocabularies.

Jack's response to a creative movement task shows him in a new and positive light

Jack, an 11-year-old boy with Aspergers syndrome, attends a mainstream recreational dance program. Jack is often difficult to manage in class, as he finds it hard to concentrate when there is a lot of noise and action in the large studio space. He is sometimes disruptive, responding at inappropriate times and more loudly than other children. However, on one occasion, a Laban-approach task that required a creative response enabled Jack to use his unusual thinking style to come up with a novel and funny solution.

continued

67

Students were asked to imagine they were holding a bowling ball and to create movements their bodies would make as they bowled, weighed down by it. After initial experimentation, Jack created a scene in which he imagined that his fingers had been superglued into the ball. His demonstration of the unexpected impact of the momentum of the moving heavy ball attached to his stationary body was hilarious. Class teacher and students alike had an opportunity to appreciate the benefits of Jack's different way of thinking.

Working with special needs children in specialised settings

There are children for whom a more specialised approach is the most suitable because of their level of need. A dance program may be provided in a special school, or in recreational settings such as a community centre.

Issues in community settings

Community-based programs present different challenges than school-based programs because of the limited contact between the program staff and children and their families. In a school, students, teachers and families have long-term daily contact, whereas in a community program, leaders and students might only meet for an hour a week. The dance group leader therefore needs to develop strategies to successfully communicate and interact with class members, particularly those who do not have verbal language skills and are restricted in what they can share about their lives. Parents and carers are thus vital links between the group leader and the child's life outside the dance program. They are also essential in providing the support the child needs in moving into a new environment and dealing with the unfamiliar expectations of a dance class.

The challenges for children in joining a dance group

Developing new relationships, learning a new set of expectations and communicating in a new context can be challenging for children with special needs, especially for those who might still be learning basic social skills. They will need support and encouragement to help them cope with the anxieties and frustrations that are likely. Time will also be needed to establish basic principles for the dance program such as sitting and standing in a circle, moving and stopping, awareness of body parts and co-operating with a partner.

Group size

It is also important that the size of the group is suited to the needs of the children. A group that is too large can result in over-stimulation and insufficient support for each individual's needs. The outcome of this can be poor focus, frustration and lack of group cohesion.

A recommended starting point is a maximum group size of six to eight children, with an ideal ratio of three children to one support worker. For example, in a class of eight children, an ideal staffing situation would be one group leader with two support workers.

Once a group is settled into a routine, it may be possible to increase the group size or decrease the amount of support. However, if the needs of the children are compromised through such an adjustment, the group leader may need to review the situation. At BreakOut, the size of the children's group has gradually increased from four participants to ten over a period of four years. We found that our capacity was ten children working with one group leader and two support workers.

Finding the right dance group for Steve

Steve, an 8-year-old boy with Down syndrome and autism, had a strong interest in dance and music. Steve's mother, wanting to extend that interest in a social context, brought him to BreakOut to see how he would enjoy participating. Given his high support needs, as a result of his dual disabilities and his tendency to abscond, it was agreed that Steve would be accompanied to class by his own support worker.

Steve's responsiveness to music through movement was instantaneous. He twirled, galloped and held hands without prompting. However, Steve stayed in his own world as he danced and despite all efforts, resisted leaving it. When the group re-assembled after each activity, Steve would refuse to join in and stayed isolated outside the circle. His carer's efforts to get him to be part of the group only frustrated him, and his enjoyment would turn to rage. This happened repeatedly throughout the session.

The other children in the group were disturbed by Steve's reactions and wanted to know what was wrong. Their participation and the flow of the session was disrupted by his angry responses. We were pleased to discover that we could get the session flowing again if we played a popular song to which everyone, including Steve, was happy to dance.

Steve attended BreakOut classes for four weeks with no change in his frustration with group activities. The situation was discussed with his mother and carer and it was agreed that BreakOut might not be the best place for Steve. Although the group has the specific intention of catering for children with special needs, the group of ten participants was too large and well established in a routine to meet the needs of a child who preferred to be in his own world.

We felt that a smaller group of three to four children, with perhaps two support workers, would offer a child like Steve a more manageable opportunity to engage in movement and music. It may be possible for him to develop a greater awareness of others and to move towards some connection with them in a smaller group. It may also benefit him to participate in a one-to-one dance therapy program to help him develop skills of relationship within the dance context.

Working towards children's independent participation

Introduction phase

The relationship between parents (or care-givers) and dance group staff is important. It is essential that parents feel comfortable with the group leader, support workers and the program being offered. Below we have listed suggested procedures for working with new children and their parents/caregivers in community settings. These are applicable for children who are intending to be independent participants.

Week 1

The parent attends the first session with the child. This enables face-to-face contact between the parent, group leader and support workers, and is an important step in developing a trusting relationship and open communication.

The parent participates in the session to gain a better understanding of the program offered and its suitability for their child. We prefer that parents actively participate rather than sit and watch, as children are more likely to be distracted by the presence of an audience. Active participation also provides a fuller experience of the dance session and the challenges for participants.

After Week 1

The parent/caregiver then evaluates the child's experience of the session. Some children may need to participate in three or four sessions before parents/carers can judge how beneficial the program might be for them.

Week 2 or 3

The parents/carers, child and group leader discuss what the goals for the child's participation in the program might be. These might be as simple as enjoyment, or may include physical exercise, social interaction or improvement of posture, co-ordination and motor skills. This is a good time for the group leader to get information about the child's interests and favourite music that could be incorporated into the dance program.

Moving towards independence

When the parent and child have made a commitment to the dance program, the next step is to taper off the parent's involvement. The process might go like this:

◉   When the child is ready to participate in the group independently, the parent should bring their child to the dance session, settle them into the room and assist with removing shoes, coats, etc, then say goodbye and leave.

◉   If a child needs support through the initial stages of settling into a group then it is advisable that the parent stay with the child and participate as an active member of the group. This can be a very useful process as the parent can demonstrate strategies for effective communication with their child. However, it is important that the parent does not stay with the child for longer than the child needs them, so that the child has the opportunity to develop independence. At BreakOut we have found that a term (10 weeks) is generally the longest amount of time that a new participant needs to be supported by a parent. Mostly separation happens more quickly.

Flora's mum supports her through the new experience of dance class

Flora and her mother Lanie visited BreakOut at the suggestion of Flora's schoolteacher who had noticed her enjoyment of music and dance. Six-year-old Flora, who has autism, had minimal verbal communication at this time. Lanie actively participated in the first BreakOut session with Flora, and gently prompted her to attend to the class. At the end of that session, Lanie expressed her delight at Flora's obvious enjoyment of the music and dance activities. Together, we then decided that it would be ideal for Lanie to continue participating while Flora familiarised herself with the activities and structure of the dance session. This would limit the number of new things Flora would need to process as a new member to the group. Lanie could also help us to develop strategies for good communication with Flora and to eliminate unnecessary frustration. For five weeks, Lanie came along as a group member and worked quietly alongside her daughter. By the sixth week, Lanie sat at the side of the room and encouraged Flora to participate independently. At this stage, I (Jenny), as the group leader, had established a good rapport with Flora and could engage her attention as well as prompt her when her attention wandered. Lanie had been a very good model, which I was thankful for once I began working on my own with Flora. By the eighth week Lanie stayed for the welcome song, then left Flora to participate independently in the group. At the beginning of the following term, Flora was very happy to see her mother leave as soon as the group assembled. Lanie has enjoyed a cup of coffee with another mother during dance time ever since.

Exceptions to the procedure: High support children

Children with high support needs are more likely to need a care-giver in attendance all the time, unless the staffing capacity of the group extends to one-to-one support. It will also be necessary to assess whether a program for children who can work independently will be suitable for a child with high support needs. It may be that a high-needs child would benefit significantly from interaction with such a group, or, on the other hand, that the group's dynamic could become fractured in aiming to meet more complex needs. A special group for children with high support needs may be a better alternative. Such assessments need to be worked out with care and sensitivity to the individual and the group.

Special occasions for care-givers

When children are participating independently, it is important to provide opportunities for families to appreciate their youngster's progress. These could take the form of a special session for families and children to dance together, an in-class presentation or a performance. Such opportunities help keep parents aware of and involved in their child's development while also nurturing the child's independence.

Sample lesson plan for children 4–8 years

Duration: 45 minutes

Preparation

Time: 15 minutes prior to starting time

- Clear the space of any obstacles or equipment that will be distracting or dangerous.
- Using a quiet, firm voice, ask children to quietly to remove their shoes and socks, coats, bags, etc. and leave outside the dance space, perhaps in the foyer or hallway.
- Play calming music as children enter the room.

Gathering and saying hello

Time: 5–7 minutes

Begin the session with all children sitting in a circle on the floor. If children have difficulty making a circle, the group leader can pre-set a circle by marking it on the floor with masking tape or by setting out a cushion for each child.

Hello song

Aim
To assemble the group and greet each child. One idea we use:

Description
 'I see you, do you?'
 'Yes I do!'
 'Can you do what I do? Name.'

The group sings these words and claps at the same time. When it comes to 'Name', the leader chooses a person in the circle by saying their name. For example: 'I see you, do you? Yes, I do! Can you do what I do? Emily…'

On hearing her name, Emily is cued to create a movement, e.g. stamping her feet. The group watches and then repeats the movement with Emily. The verse is repeated around the circle, allowing each child to have a turn.

Warm-up

Time: 10 minutes
Choose two of these options

Moving and stopping

Aim
To warm up the body, develop focus and body control.

Description

Group leader gives the cue to begin moving by playing music (recorded or percussion instrument such as a drum, shaker or tambourine). The cue to stop moving is when the music stops.

Variation

Children accompany movement with small handshakers (maraccas), playing as they move and stopping when they stop.

or

Moving and stopping in shapes

Aim

To continue warm-up and add spatial awareness challenges.

Equipment

Masking tape, simple percussion instruments such as handshakers.

Description

Mark out shapes on the floor with masking tape, such as circles, triangles, stars or squares. Shapes need to be big enough for two to three people to stand inside.

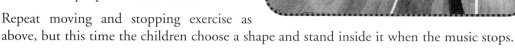

Repeat moving and stopping exercise as above, but this time the children choose a shape and stand inside it when the music stops.

Variation

This activity can be developed into a way of teaching children how to make group shapes with body parts. Repeat the exercise as above and when children stop in their chosen shape the group leader nominates a body part, e.g. hands and children within the shape connect by touching hands. This can be repeated using different body parts.

Music

Something lively and energetic such as:

- John Paul Young, *Strictly Ballroom* soundtrack, 'Love Is In The Air'.
- Various artists (2000) *Children's Party*, Musicband Ltd, Volume 2.

Teaching tip

Remove masking tape from the floor after the session. It is very difficult to remove from polished floors as it ages. Eucalyptus oil is useful for removing traces.

Moving and stopping with the drum

Aim
Continue warm-up as above, and add leadership skills.

Equipment
Drum, cushions and chairs.

Description
Place a combination of cushions and chairs around the floor, spread well apart. A selected child or group of children play the drums. All move when the drum plays and stop by sitting on chairs or cushions when the drum stops. The different heights of chairs and cushions brings in the use of different levels in space.

Animal soup

Aim
To warm up body parts engage imagination and develop connection between imaginative play and movement.

Description
The group leader sets up an imaginary bowl of soup (perhaps in an inverted drum) and explains that it is full of magical soup that will help everyone dance, because it is made up of animals. Each child chooses an animal and demonstrates how that animal moves. The movements, for example, galloping, sliding, walking tall, stomping or crawling are then put into the soup. The inclusion of animals with contrasting movements, such as a horse and a snake or a cat and an elephant can be encouraged. The whole group then use their hands to 'stir' the soup and take a big drink, cupping the imaginary soup in their hands. After tasting the soup, one child can nominate the kind of soup it is, and the class begins the 'animal dance' by exploring the movements of the named animal. After each movement, the group can return to the soup bowl for another drink and new movement/animal. To bring the exercise to an end, the group can return to the bowl of soup and shake out all the animals.

Music
Something lively such as Various artists (1999), *World Playground*, Putumayo Music.

Skill Development

Time: 10 minutes

Choose one of these activities.

Rolling, crawling and jumping

Aim
Progression through developmental movement patterns at different levels.

Equipment
Two long pieces of fabric approximately 6 metres long and small hand scarves.

Description

Place long piece of fabric (approximately 6 metres) on the floor.

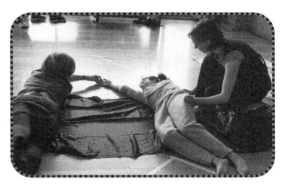

- *Rolling:* One by one children lie on fabric on their backs and roll down the fabric as far as they can go.
- *Crawling:* Group leader and assistant create a tunnel by holding a piece of fabric over the fabric on the floor. Children crawl along fabric through the tunnel.
- *Jumping:* Fabric is positioned across the width of the room on the floor. Children take turns to leap over the fabric in pairs or as a group all holding hands. Begin with the fabric folded fairly narrow and gradually widen it as children master jumping.

Variation

To encourage the use of the arms, children can hold small scarves in their hands. The image of a bird flying with outstretched wings could be suggested.

Music

Something flowing and mellow such as Vann Tiersen (2001) *Amelie* soundtrack, Track 4.

Tightrope walk

Aims

To develop focus, balance and co-ordination.

Equipment

Masking tape, or length of ribbon and small umbrellas.

Description

Create a line along the length of the floor with masking tape or a length of ribbon taped to floor. Children walk the length of the tape, placing one foot carefully in front of the other as if they are walking along a tightrope.

Variations

- *Circus umbrella:* A small umbrella is a good prop to help engage the imagination for this activity and to encourage the use of the upper body.
- *Relay game:* The group can be divided into two, so that one child starts and walks to the other end, then passes the umbrella to the next child, just like passing the baton in a relay race, until everyone has had a turn.

Music

Something magical, stately and flowing such as:

- Cirque du Soleil, *Collections*, Track 3
- K.C. Wang (1996), *Chinese Bamboo Flute Songs*, Track 1.

Time to dance!

Time: 15 – 20 minutes

Choose two or three of these activities.

Galloping

Aim

Co-ordination, rhythm through movement, co-operating with partner, directional movement, aerobic exercise.

Description

Children stand behind one another, lengthwise down the side of the room. The group leader faces them and leads galloping sideways across the room and back to the starting position.

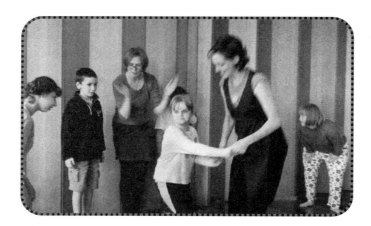

Variations

- ◎ *Children clap hands as they gallop:* Start as above. After children complete their first set of gallops across the room, they stop and begin a clapping sequence, e.g. hands clap on thighs and then together. Repeat clapping sequence a few times before galloping across to the other side.

- ◎ *Galloping with partner:* Each child holds hands with a partner. Encourage eye contact by saying, 'Can you see your partner's face?' Gallop across the room facing your partner.

- ◎ *Galloping with partner and clapping:* Gallop across room with partner. Stop at the other side and begin clapping sequence, e.g. clap hands together, then clap hands with partner.

Music

The group leader can beat out a gallop rhythm with rhythm sticks, or lively jig such as

- ◎ Hot Toddy (1999) *Celtic Fire*
- ◎ Jugularity (1996) *Greatest Hits*, Tracks 5 and 7.

Ribbon dancing

Aims

To extend movement through arms, develop movement flow, spatial awareness and decision-making.

Equipment

A basket full of colourful ribbons approximately 1.5 metres long

Description

Each child chooses a ribbon from a basket and finds a place to stand in their own space in the room. The group leader asks the children, 'What can your ribbon do?', then initiates experimentation with some of the following ideas:

◎ *Shape:* Circles in the air, circle on the floor, wiggly lines.

◎ *Movement:* Throwing ribbon high into the air, walking slowly with the ribbon trailing behind on the ground or rocking side to side with ribbon stretched out over the head.

◎ *Connection:* Moving close to a group member so that ribbons touch and move together. The whole group can come together to touch ribbons before moving back to 'your own space'.

Music

Something flowing and lively such as:

◎ Hi 5 (2001) *Jump and Jive with Hi 5*, Track 7.

◎ Various artists, (2000) *Children's Party*, Volume 2

Create your own circle dance

Description

Each child takes it in turn to be the leader by stepping into the middle of the circle and creating their own movement. The group follows the movement. When the child is finished they step back into the circle and the next child steps in to the centre until everyone has had a turn being the leader. It may take a while before every child feels confident to lead. Positive feedback will help.

Music

This activity provides the perfect opportunity for children to select their own music. Use a different child's favourite music each session.

Folk dance:

Music

Use a familiar song that has well-known actions for the group to enjoy singing and dancing together.

◎ Recordings such as David Moses (1994) *Okki Tokki Unga*
Various artists (1998), *The Bird Dance And Other Party Favourites*

◎ Some examples are 'Hokey Pokey' or 'Lobby Loo'.

Relaxation and goodbye

Time: 5–10 minutes
Choose one of these

Soft wave

Aims
To calm the mind and relax the body.

Equipment
Two pieces of long fabric (4–5 metres)

Description
Children lie side by side on fabric. Using a second piece of fabric of similar length, the teacher and assistant create a soft 'wave' over the top of the children. The 'wave' gently touches the children's body and then lifts again.

Massage

Equipment
Big basket, fabric squares 1 metre x 1 metre in a variety of colours; soft brushes, e.g. make-up or shaving brushes.

Description
Each child chooses a piece of fabric from the basket and places it on the floor in their own special spot. The child then lies on the fabric and the group leader covers each one with a 'blanket' made of another piece of fabric. The group leader moves from child to child giving each one a foot or hand massage using hands or a soft brush.

Music
Something calm, slow and soothing such as:
◎   Baby Bach, (2000) *babyeinsteinmusic,* Tracks 10 and 11

Goodbye song

Aims
To reassemble as a group after relaxation, reactivate a level of alertness and bring the session to an end.

Description
Each member is farewelled by group leader and members with a song:

> *'Good bye* **'Name'***,*
>
> *Goodbye* **'Name'***,*
>
> *Goodbye* **'Name'**
>
> *Thanks for dancing today'.*

Sample lesson plan for children
8–12 years (suitable for those with and without special needs)

The lesson detailed below is based on a 45-minute session with 25 children. It is possible to make a session shorter or longer to suit the group or school's schedule, but the elements of warm-up, and relaxation/cool-down must be included, even if in a reduced form.

An ideal ratio of students to staff in a group that includes a child or children with disabilities would be, in addition to the teacher, one aide for each special needs child. In practice this may not occur, so a teacher must be prepared to cope with a range of abilities and responses to any given tasks.

Preparation

Time: 15 minutes prior to starting time

- ◎ Clear the space of any obstacles or equipment that will be distracting or dangerous.
- ◎ Using a quiet, firm voice, ask children to quietly to remove their shoes and socks, coats, bags, etc. and leave outside the dance space, perhaps in the foyer or hallway.
- ◎ Play calming music as children enter the room.

Welcome

Greet children and ask them to sit close to you on the floor. Welcome them to the dance/movement program and briefly explain the plan for the session.

Time: 5 minutes

Introductory song

(Optional – suitable for small groups of children up to about 8 years).

Description
Children sit in a circle.

Use a song to greet each member of the class, but only if the session is at least 60 minutes long, and the group small. For younger children in a small group, this is a way to help a teacher learn the name of each child and to greet each one individually. It also encourages confident use of voice from class members.

A greeting song might go like this. The class sings:

'Sing us your name,
Sing us your name,
Sing us your name,
That's the game.'

(Shenanigans, 1989, 'Sing Me Your Name', from *There's A Wombat in My Room*

Child responds: *My name is Kim, that's my name.*

Class echoes: *Your name is Kim, that's your name.*

For children who have difficulty singing solo, the teacher or another student might accompany them. The class can keep the beat by tapping on their knees.

Warm-up

Time: 10 minutes

Move and freeze

Aim
Children must be able to handle their own movements enough to stop when requested. This helps the teacher to stay in control and to keep the space safe. This activity is enjoyed by both boys and girls, and can be successfully undertaken by any child who can co-operate and follow verbal instructions.

Description
Children move through the space, stopping when given the instruction 'Freeze!'. 'Move and freeze' introduces the basic 'effort' elements of dance: Weight, Space, Flow and Time (described in Chapter 2). There are many ways to vary this activity. An element of surprise will ensure that children listen carefully.

Music dynamics
Changing the dynamics of the musical accompaniment will have a strong impact on the elicited movement.

- *Rhythm:* for example, skip (double beat), gallop, triplet, waltz.
  - *Gallop*: double beat with a strong emphasis on the second beat.
  - *Triplet:* 3/4 time with even beats.
  - *Waltz:* 3/4 time with emphasis on first beat.

- *Vary length of phrase:* Short or long phrases, and a variety, e.g. playing one very short phrase between a series of long ones.
- *Change volume:* Begin with strong beats to ensure children can hear clearly in the chaos of a busy room. Then change to lighter (quieter beats) and a combination of these.
- *Change tempo:* Intersperse quick tempo beats with slower ones.

Movement repertoire
- *Change direction:* Forwards, backwards, sideways, diagonally, in circles, backwards (best done slowly), or combinations.
- *Change level:* High, medium, low, along the floor.
- *Combinations:* Moving forwards quickly could be followed by moving backwards slowly.
- *Change movements used: (continued)*

Give instructions such as:

- 'No walking or running allowed this time. Find a different way to move!'
- 'Only one leg is allowed to touch the floor as you travel.'
- 'Find a way to move backwards and low.'

Different ways to 'freeze'

Body shapes

◉   Focus on body parts: 'When you freeze, only hands and knees may touch the floor'. 'Only bottoms allowed to touch the floor.'

◉   Focus on levels: 'Freeze making a high shape / in a shape that is very close to the floor.'

◉   Focus on shape: 'Make a shape that looks like you have been twisted.'

Working with a partner

◉   Move in groups of three, all moving the same way.

◉   Move with partner, both moving the same way, but one high and one low.

◉   Move with one other person, someone you haven't worked with already today (a great way to get new ideas and combinations).

◉   When you freeze, make a group of four people.

◉   Freeze with a partner, touching by elbows only.

Music

Drum accompaniment. A hand drum like an Irish Bodhran, tambour or small African djembe with a shoulder strap is ideal so that the teacher can vary the beat and tempo to challenge students.

Travel patterns

Time: 10 minutes

Run, jump, run

Aim

This activity has worked for me in every classroom I (Kim) have been in, even with the most unenthusiastic and inexperienced participants. It is very simple and uses basic pedestrian movements, so that no one can get it wrong. It also accommodates children with a range of abilities and allows them to gradually extend their experimentation as their confidence builds. It is usually played from corner to corner of the room, allowing the most distance for travelling.

Description

The teacher models the sequence of movements: run, jump and run finishing with a freeze. Children then try this sequence, one by one across the space. Once the basic sequence of movements is mastered, children create their own sequence of a run, a jump and run and then finish with a freeze.

Each child creates his/her own moves as well as observing the ideas of the rest of their class.

Variations

Change moving words

As the class masters the initial activity, the teacher can change the 'moving' words, for example, to 'skip, spin, slide'. To ensure that everyone, including children with disabilities understand the meaning of these words, you can:

- ask a class member to define the suggested movement, i.e.
  'Who can describe what a "slide" is?'
- ask a class member to demonstrate their version of the new movement, e.g.
  'Who can show me what a "spin" is?'
- add only one new concept at a time, e.g. 'run, jump, run' can become 'run, spin, run', then 'run, spin, slide', then 'skip, spin, slide'
- give each person an opportunity to practise in their own space before putting the three movements together as they travel
- reinforce that there is no right or wrong way to do this activity. Each person's response is equally valuable. Sometimes an idea will work as planned, at other times it won't, but the point is to try!

Working with others

Extend this activity further by adding the complication of working with others. Children can be asked to choose one or more other people to work with. The first time, the leader can ask them to choose their own partner/s. The next time, they can be asked to extend beyond their close friends by being asked to 'choose someone you haven't worked with today'. Ideas for partner work include:

- travelling together making the same movements
- travelling together making different kinds of the same movements (e.g. one walks forwards while the other walks backwards) and finish at the same time
- find a new way to move, e.g. one or two children may leapfrog over another to make a new kind of 'jump'
- travel in canon (see glossary), one following the next.

Music

Sidney Berlin Ragtime Band and others (1994) *Doop Doop*.

This music always draws a favourable response from children as it is uptempo, fun and interesting, yet has a regular beat.

Theme

Time: 10 minutes

Creative movement response to a story or poem

Aims

One way to extend movement exploration skills is the creation of a choreography. This can be as simple as a class activity, or focused on the development of a performance. Stories provide a great starting point for creative choreographies for children. The choice of a story that allows for difference in movements, abilities and interests, provides all students with the possibility of a successful interpretation.

Description

Creating a choreography from a story: Begin by reading the story aloud to the class. Children discuss their favourite characters and parts of the story, prompted by such question as 'What part of the story did you like best? Why was that the best part?'

For example, if you were reading the line from Lewis Carroll's nonsense poem *Jabberwocky*: 'T'was brilling and the slithy toves', you might ask:

> 'What is brilling? How would it feel? What would it look like?'

> 'What are toves? What is a shape that a tove might make? When a tove moves in a slithy way, what would it look like?'

Children then experiment with movements associated with those sections or characters of the story. Interesting and unusual responses can be shared with the whole class. For example;

> 'David, the way you slithered so low along the ground looked very interesting. Could you show the class how you did it?'

David demonstrates.

> 'Now, let's see if everyone can make themselves as low and slithy a Tove as David did. Does anyone have another idea about how slithy looks – something that is different from David's?'

Then the ideas can be connected into a choreography.

Music

Mortal Combat, *Mortal Combat* movie soundtrack.

Relaxation and farewell

Time: 5 to 10 minutes

Relaxation

Aim

To settle students after the dance session, in readiness for classroom desk work. If students regularly return from dance classes so energised that they cannot co-operate in their next class, classroom teachers' enthusiasm for the dance program will soon wane.

Description

The relaxation ideas from Chapter 2 that require the least amount of individual teacher input are suitable for use with large classroom-sized groups. 'Flying Wave' is such an activity, but it requires the assistance of an aide or helpful student.

Variation

A variation of the 'Flying Wave' is the 'Flying Bird'.

The teacher holds a flying bird puppet and walks slowly around the room, allowing the bird to fly down and land for a moment on children who are lying quietly and still. The concern about missing out on a visit from the bird will provide strong motivation for children who find it difficult to settle.

For children who need a little extra assistance to relax, the teacher or aide can provide some focused encouragement by placing a firm hand on the forehead or sternum (if child lies on their back) or small of the back of the child (if the child lies on their stomach) and sitting quietly beside the student until they have settled.

Music
Something soothing and calming such as:

◎ Howlin' Wind, (1995) *Dugong Lullaby*, Track 6 'Starfish Lagoon'

Farewell

Description
When the bird has visited everyone, children can be asked to slowly wake up.

Instructions to ensure a quiet and orderly wake-up
◎ Slowly roll over onto your side, then come up onto your feet. See if you can do it as quietly as the bird flew.
◎ Stretch your wings out wide to the side, then up above your head.
◎ Bring your wings down by your side again, making them reach as far out to the side as you can as they come down.
◎ Try this again and this time, breathe right in and let your wings lift you right up onto your toes.
◎ As you let your breath out of your body, let your wings and then your whole body drop forward over your knees.
◎ Slowly come to a standing position as you breathe in again.
◎ Let your wings change back into arms and give your whole body a small shake all-over.

Variation
For groups who need more assistance to stay settled, children can be asked to go and quietly put on their shoes and socks one by one after they have been visited by the bird.

Feedback and discussion

Finish by thanking the children for their hard work and co-operation for the session. If there is time, you might ask for feedback from one or two class members about what they enjoyed most during the session and what they might like to do the next time. Then briefly summarise the session's activities and give a brief overview of what the class will be doing in the next session. Include a reminder about any 'homework' students might have for the next time (e.g. bringing in a favourite piece of music to dance to, thinking of some new movement ideas or words for 'Run, jump run', choosing the people to work with for the choreography).

More ideas

The ideas suggested for dance class activities in Chapter 2 are also appropriate for working with children.

How to choose a suitable story

There are hundreds of possible stories. Important issues for the selection of stories that provide good stimuli for creative dance are:

- ◉ Are the characters interesting?
- ◉ What do they do? How do they move? (If the book doesn't tell us, can we work it out ourselves?)
- ◉ Are there enough parts for everyone in the class?
- ◉ Do the illustrations help the class get inspired?

Two stories I have used successfully with students are

- ◉ *Where the Wild Things Are* by Maurice Sendak (suitable for children approx. 4–8 years)
- ◉ *Jabberwocky,* nonsense poem by Lewis Carroll (suitable for children approx. 8 years and over), from *Alice in Wonderland.*

> Twas brilling and the slithy toves
> Did gyre and gimble in the wabe
> All mimsy were the borogoves
> And the mome rath outgabe
> Beware the Jabberwock my son
> The jaws that bite, the claws that snatch
> Beware the Jub Jub bird and shun
> The frumious bandersnatch

Jabberwocky is ideal for integrated groups of slightly older children because it allows for different ways of thinking. Because there is no absolute meaning for many of these words there can be no absolute right or wrong answer. Children who have sophisticated language comprehension and vocabulary might be challenged by thinking of alliterative qualities of words, such as the relationship between slithy and 'real' words such as slithery and slimy. Others who have less mastery of language may be able to respond in a bodily way, to show their response to the word or concept in movement. Whether or not they grasp the language concepts in the same way as the more sophisticated thinkers doesn't prevent them from having a valid response, which may be no less interesting or creative.

This process of responding to stories in movement requires no formal skills or muscle memory of movements, such as, for example, a jazz routine would, and can be achieved by people who do not have good verbal communication. Sometimes, this activity provides a new view of a student, abilities not seen in other contexts, as demonstrated by the following story of Tom:

Tom and the Tum Tum Tree

In a primary school, a class of Grade 5 students and I (Kim) were creating a Laban-based choreography for a performance. Tom, a large strong boy who had learning disabilities and ADHD, really struggled to co-operate with the other students. Consequently, he had difficulty socially and his classmates often preferred to leave him out of groups they selected for dance activities. Tom found this frustrating, but also knew that he would quickly reach the limit of his tolerance and capacity for negotiation when trying to work closely physically with others to explore an idea.

In the creation of the dance piece, *Jabberwocky*, based on Lewis Carroll's poem, all students selected their own characters. The text of the poem is made up of nonsense words, so students were free to create their own manifestations of the characters, including movements, physical appearance and interaction with others.

Tom made a marvellous choice for himself as the Tum Tum Tree. His size and strength were perfect for the role and provided an imposing visual focal point for the whole choreography. Tom was able to develop his own character, choreograph his simple movements and costume himself with only a minimum of input from staff. His simple costume was devised out of a piece of brown fabric that he found in the schools dress-up box. As he had mastery over his own role, he was happy to co-operate sufficiently with the Son and the Jabberwock characters to create an interaction that delighted them all and suitably portrayed the dramatic story. Tom managed the final performance, his first time in a solo role, with alacrity. His class teacher was particularly delighted with his achievement, given Tom's less than successful record of contributions to group events with this class.

With continuing experiences of success, like that of his performance of the Tum Tum Tree, Tom and other students would hopefully develop a more positive sense of him and his capacities. The next time around, Tom might even be successful as part of a co-operative group process.

Poem: Lewis Carroll, *Jabberwocky*, from *Alice in Wonderland*

Further reading

Inclusive physical education classrooms:

Block, M. (2000) *A teacher's guide to including students with disabilities in general physical education* 2ed. Brookes: Maryland.

Movement and dance with young children who have special needs

Guthrie, J. and Roydhouse, J. (1988), *Come and Join The Dance*, Hyland House: Melbourne

Stinson, S. (1988), *Dance for Young Children: Finding The Magic in Movement*, AAPERD: Virginia.

Chapter 4

Working with adults

Working with groups that include people of different abilities

People with intellectual disabilities who attend schools, day training centres and recreational activities are usually grouped according to their support needs. People with high support needs are usually in a group with others who require the same level of care and co-active assistance. People with more independent skills also tend to be grouped together. In most centres this is a very clear distinction, as it enables a better quality of service to be delivered.

However, there are times when a group leader faces a group that includes people with different and even contradictory needs. These challenges are sometimes more pronounced with groups that are comprised of people with more independent skills. Individual behavioural issues and idiosyncrasies will often present themselves in more immediate ways in such groups. I (Jenny) have found many challenges running a program for young adults at an adult training service. While all members of this group are considered 'independent', there is a challenging range of needs to be accommodated. Some members have the need for very firm boundaries to help them deal with emotional distress, some need the freedom to come and go from the program because of their autism or difficulty with group participation, while others need to be directed back to the group because of their difficulty in maintaining focus. There is also the challenge of working with a diverse range of abilities. In this same group of young adults there are members who have a strong connection with their bodies and the ability to move in an expressive way and those who are more reserved in their use of their body or who are physically restricted.

It can also be challenging to lead a program that includes people who do not want to be part of the group. This can happen despite the very best intentions of the management of a centre. This is one challenge that could be eliminated to the benefit of all involved by discussing the situation with the program co-ordinator. It is a misconception often held about people with intellectual disabilities that involvement in anything is good for them. It is vital to the functioning of a dance program that participants want to be part of the action and are at least motivated enough to engage to some degree. It is important that a person's determined lack of engagement is respected.

Community-based groups like BreakOut, which participants attend voluntarily in their own free time also face these challenges, but generally not to the same degree. At BreakOut, new volunteers and visitors often comment on the high level of focus evident in the groups. We have always attributed this to the fact that members attend BreakOut by choice and that they enjoy being part of the group and the experience of dancing. Parents and carers often tell us about excitement and anticipation in their homes the night before classes. Yet even with this level of motivation there are still challenges associated with responding to different needs and abilities within the groups.

Strategies for working with groups of people with different needs and abilities

The group leader should aim to lead a program that will include all members as well as providing opportunities for exploration of new movements and ideas, especially for those people who are more independent.

Developing focus

The first 10 to 15 minutes of the session should be devoted to activities that focus the group and develop interaction between members. These are best done with participants sitting on chairs in a circle. They include:

- name games
- passing a ball or balloon between members of the group
- catching bubbles
- giant elastic (see Chapter 5 on Props)
- following the movement of a designated leader
- musical chairs (without eliminations)
- swapping chairs (see Chapter 2)
- following movements of a designated leader and passing on leadership around the circle. Even the simplest movement and response from a participant can be acknowledged and used as a stimulus for the group to follow.

Moving through space

A dance session should include a section in which all members move through the space. If group members are ambulant, all chairs can be put away. If some members need chairs, they can be positioned so that they do not obstruct the flow of movement around the room, but so that people sitting on them can see what is happening. Ideas for moving around the space can include:

- walking with a partner and, when the music stops, changing partners
- walking with partner and, when the music stops, the name of a body part is called out by the group leader and partners make a shape connecting with that body part. (See Chapter 3 for other ideas for this activity.)

Support from assistants

The leader should direct support workers to assist group members who find it difficult to maintain focus and social interaction. This will help them to engage in the exercise, which in turn will help the group maintain focus. The support worker should begin by standing or sitting next to the person, then

- quietly verbally prompt and encourage them
- gently co-actively assist them with the activity
- support them with 'time-out' from the group if participation becomes too difficult.

This does not mean coercing or forcing a group member to participate in an activity. While encouragement is appropriate, force is not.

Coping with withdrawal

A group leader needs to develop a strategy that accommodates people who find it difficult to stay in the room for extended periods of time. The leader is responsible for the safety of all participants, so it is important that they acknowledge when a group member needs to take time-out and ensure they are adequately supervised. A good strategy is for the group leader to continue with the program in order to maintain the focus of other group members, while a designated support worker accompanies the person for some time-out.

If a group member has decided to withdraw from an exercise and sit to the side, it is important to acknowledge this choice. Sometimes they may only need a little encouragement to rejoin the group, for example, by the group leader offering to partner them for an activity. However, if the person has made a firm decision not to participate, then the leader can suggest that they participate as an 'audience'. Watching is a constructive form of participation, especially if the member is encouraged to offer feedback to performers.

If a participant is resisting joining the group but is comfortable about staying in the dance space, the group leader should initiate contact with that person throughout the program. This could be as simple as sitting next to the person while they explain an exercise. This draws the person back into the group without any demands. Using props such as balloons, balls and scarves provide a fun means of interaction which can be sustained for a short or long period of time. If a person responds to this type of interaction, a support worker could continue working one-to-one with the person while the group leader continues with the rest of the program.

Extending the higher functioning participants

Members who can maintain focus, and have a good capacity to express themselves through movement, need to be extended. This is one of the biggest challenges when managing a group with different abilities and needs. By structuring the session to include all members at the beginning, it is reasonable to allow 10 to15 minutes for working with material that extends the movement experience of more able members. Some of these activities, described in detail in Chapter 2, include Pushing, Pulling and Melting; Sculptor and Clay; Improvisation and Solos. If other less competent members wander during this time, the strategies listed in the previous paragraph can be used.

Providing performing opportunities for more able group members

Opportunities to perform solos or duos are a good way of extending the capabilities of each individual. Performing opportunities are very appealing to group members who really love to dance, while also accommodating those who are more restricted in their dance and movement abilities. The room can be set up as for a traditional stage/audience-style performance space with the performer at the front, or with members positioned in a large circle so that the centre becomes the performance space. Solos and duets can be a satisfying ending to a session.

Reconnecting the group at the end of the session

Returning to the circle is a good strategy to reconnect a group after it has become fragmented. Sitting on the floor or on chairs is helpful in grounding the energy of the group if people have become overexcited or agitated. Choose a focusing activity to help the group reconnect. An example of one such activity is the passing of a lighted candle around the circle.

The benefits of diversity

This section has highlighted some of the challenges of working with groups of people with intellectual disabilities. A group leader working in a day centre or recreational setting, where there is likely to be a diverse range of abilities within a group, needs to feel comfortable with these challenges. While at times it can feel very chaotic working with a diversity of needs and abilities, the rewards and benefits mostly outweigh the frustration. For example, it can be very rewarding when the more able members use their skills to assist the less able in the group, or when a person who is very withdrawn watches a performance with a big smile on their face. However, if you are a group leader who would prefer to work with a group who all share the same level of motivation, so that together you can develop as dancers and performers, it would be better to set up a group specifically for that purpose.

Enjoy the diversity!

Working with older adults

The benefits of participation in dance for older adults

People with intellectual disabilities are often much less fit, active and healthy than other adults in the community, so a program comprised of adults who are 40 years and over might be considered an older adult group. Often the challenge for a group leader working with older adults who have intellectual disabilities is to engage, and keep them engaged, in program activities. Older adults with intellectual disabilities are much less likely to cause themselves injury or discomfort through exertion than other older adults. However, the following information is included to help ensure the safety of all participants, especially those who do apply themselves to the dance program with energy and enthusiasm.

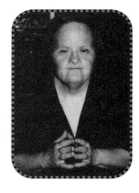

Physical benefits

Research has indicated the benefits of regular physical activity for older adults including important positive effects on the musculoskeletal, cardiovascular, respiratory and endocrine systems (US Surgeon-General, 1996; WHO, 1997). Exercise reduces the risk of coronary heart disease, hypertension, colon cancer, diabetes mellitus and early death. Many of the conditions specifically associated with older age can be impacted positively by involvement in physical exercise. Flexibility exercises can reduce the tightness and stiffness in the joints of arthritis sufferers. Weight-bearing activities benefit people with osteoporosis by increasing bone mass. Simply standing for several minutes at a time has been shown to slightly increase bone mass in people with severe osteoporosis. For people with Parkinson's disease, a program that incorporates flexibility and balance exercises and relaxation can extend muscle tightness, improve balance and reduce tremors.

Psychological, social and cultural benefits

Physical exercise also has psychological benefits, including reduction in depression and anxiety, improved mood and enhancement of the ability to perform daily tasks throughout the life span (US Surgeon-General, 1996). Programs that are carried out in small groups and/or social environments also enhance social and intercultural interactions for many older adults (WHO, 1997).

With regard to people with dementia, dance therapist Heather Hill suggests that 'dance has much to offer in terms of meeting not only physical but also social and emotional needs' (2001, p. 1). The experience of dance can provide a means for family members to connect with their relatives who have dementia through an enjoyable shared activity. Other benefits include a physical release, a chance to connect to memories and feelings, acquire more positive feelings about one's body and self, and the opportunity for group members to nurture each other. Hill also describes the value of dance experience for care staff who 'enjoy seeing residents in a different state of being. The opportunity to see behind the mask of dementia … the time and the space to relate to residents simply as human being to human being' (2001, p. 1).

Attributes needed for working with older adults

A leader of a group for older adults with disabilities needs to have a good sense of humour, patience and a non-hurried approach. The leader must be prepared to allow group members plenty of time in their responses to facilitate the highest level of functioning that the combined impacts of age and disability will allow. For many older adults with intellectual disabilities, especially those who have been institutionalised, the challenges of creative thinking and physical exertion can be fairly overwhelming.

The leader must have an appropriate energy level: high enough to be able to inspire and sustain the group, without being too exhausting. It can be tricky finding the right balance of attunement between the generally lower energy level of older adults and the high level of energy usually needed for motivating leadership. The following case example describes the challenges of trying to involve Marg, a woman in her sixties with Down syndrome, in the activities of the older adult group at BreakOut. A very patient approach, continuing encouragement and repetition of favoured activities were the strategies that eventually assisted Marg to participate happily.

Marg slowly finds her way to enjoying new experiences in the dance program

Marg first came to BreakOut sessions when another resident from her home began to attend. Marg had made the choice to attend the group, but spent much of each session in tears, huddled comfortlessly against the wall of the hall. Occasionally she could be cajoled into joining in with an activity, but as soon as that changed or a new activity was introduced, she would begin to cry all over again. We decided to try and help Marg enjoy sessions more by focusing on activities that she was comfortable with and keeping new activities to a minimum. After many weeks of experimenting and careful observation of Marg's responses, we gradually began to figure out the activities that we could successfully involve her in and those that she found too stressful.

Gradually we began to make progress and Marg's confidence and enjoyment increased. Week by week she became more active in class, sometimes leading a game or activity with a cheeky grin or a laugh. Marg often had interesting ideas when it was time for improvisation, and she really enjoyed activities in which she could work with a partner, especially when that person was co-operative. It was hard to reconcile this new Marg with our memory of the unhappy woman who had come to BreakOut two years earlier.

General safety guidelines for older adults

These guidelines have mostly been adapted from Clark (1998). This reference is recommended for people seeking more detailed information.

- Err on the side of safety at all times.
- Progress should be slow and gradual.
- Ensure that breath continues evenly throughout exercises.
- Any activity that causes pain should be modified or stopped immediately.
- Do not over-bend or over-stretch the joints.
- Limit overhead arm work.
- Perform moves that involve turning or bending the back separately, rather than combining the two.
- Use caution with neck activities. Do not move the neck quickly. Avoid nodding very low, and tilting backwards of the head.
- Limit turning and spinning, and keep the tempo slow.
- Temperature: Keep the dance space at a comfortable temperature. As a person ages, their body becomes more sensitive to heat and cold, and it is more difficult to retain or dissipate heat. In hot weather, encourage frequent water breaks and ensure adequate ventilation.
- Older adults should never dance after eating a large meal, as there is a slightly increased risk of heart attack. They should wait for at least one hour, ideally two, after a large meal.

Asthma

- Warm-ups and cool-downs are especially important for people with asthma. A 15-minute warm-up allows the respiratory system to adapt and helps prevent asthma episodes.
- Some older adults with asthma have difficulty moving for extended periods. Short, intermittent bouts of exercise may be more effective than one long bout. Once the participant becomes accustomed to the program, the duration of exercise can gradually be increased.
- Extremely cold temperatures can make asthma symptoms worse.
- If a participant has any shortness of breath, they should stop and rest until they are comfortable.
- End each session with cool-down activities that include a stretch and relaxation.

Dementia or Alzheimer's disease

People with Down syndrome are particularly susceptible to Alzheimer's disease, which often occurs 20 to 25 years earlier than in the general population (Dalton 1995).

Simple repetitive activities are appropriate. Part of the focus of a dance program for people with dementia is to engage them. Provide lots of verbal praise and positive reinforcement.

Mornings are a better time for a dance program, when participants are less fatigued.

Later stages of dementia

People with Alzheimer's sometimes have angry outbursts and display physical aggression. These acts of aggression may occur randomly and will only last a few minutes. This behaviour is part of the disease and has nothing to do with the leader or the program. The person often doesn't even understand what they are saying. If a participant is disruptive, remove them from the group until they calm down. Memory loss becomes more pronounced during the later stages.

- The participant's care-giver may need to be present during the dance session to provide familiarity.
- It is important to provide a structured program with little variation for a client in the later stages of such a cognitive disorder. An introduction to new activities may confuse them.
- Never leave a participant with Alzheimer's alone as they are likely to wander off.
- More information about working with older adults with dementia can be found in Heather Hill's book, *Invitation to the Dance* (2001).

Hearing impairments

- Always face the participant when you speak.
- Reduce background noise or move to a quiet area to speak to the participant.
- Keep your hands away from your face.
- Speak with a normal clear tone. Shouting will distort the sound of your voice.
- Use visual cues as often as possible in combination them with your verbal instructions.

Hypertension

- Older adults, especially those with hypertension, should avoid high-intensity exercise. Always begin dance activities at a very low intensity.

Obesity

- Obese participants are more susceptible to injury, fatigue and dehydration.

Osteoporosis

- Avoid quick, jarring movements that might lead to a fall or fracture. Avoid twisting movements.
- Be careful when performing any back exercises. If the participant complains of pain, stop the activity.
- Weight-bearing activities should not be undertaken until at least eight weeks after a hip fracture.

Parkinson's disease

- Flexibility exercises are important for people with Parkinson's, who often have a great deal of muscle tightness
- Balance is a major problem, so activities to assist with balance should be included in the dance program. However, the leader should ensure that the environment is as safe as possible and there is minimal risk of the participant falling.
- Parkinson's sufferers usually have a delay when starting a movement, so more time to initiate movement needs to be allowed.
- Breathing exercises are also important, such as the pursed lips breathing exercise described on page 97. Participants can practise expiring air (like blowing out candles) to strengthen their respiratory muscles.
- Relaxation techniques appear to be very helpful in reducing tremors.

Visual impairments

- Use brightly coloured tape (yellow or pink) to mark objects that might cause injury.
- Verbal instructions are very important for people who cannot see well.

Using chairs: The benefits and disadvantages

When working with older adults, it is important to have the option of working from a chair. While weight-bearing activities and movements in active functional positions are ideal, many older adults will not have the stamina to complete a whole session on their feet, or have the mobility or balance to manage challenging activities from a standing position. Incorporating opportunities to sit down will extend the amount of time and energy participants can expend in class. A session might include some standing activity and seated stretches, and optional standing work using the back of the chair for balance support.

For the frailest, older adults, or those with more limiting disabilities, seated exercise may be the only possible strategy. There are still great benefits to be gained from more limited programs comprised of gentle stretches, posture and breathing exercises.

Chairs without arms are preferable, as they make it easier for participants to extend their movements. However, sometimes chairs with arms are unavoidable, especially for people in wheelchairs. The program must be flexible enough to accommodate this. Ideally the participant's feet should be in full contact with the floor. A book or stool can be used for this purpose if necessary.

There are many ways to modify activities so that they can be done seated. The warm-up activities described in Chapter 2 can also be done when seated. Experiment with ways of walking and moving from a seat. A chair also provides a secure position for the use of motivating and attention-grabbing props such as scarves, elastics and balls.

Sample session for chair-bound older adults

The session detailed below is based on a 60-minute session with eight participants and two support workers. This is an ideal length of time for a session, as it does not over-stretch participants' concentration or the length of time spent in one room. With a larger group, it might be possible to extend the session to 75 minutes by extending the relaxation time. In most cases, the maximum desirable length of a session is 90 minutes. The extra time might allow for conversational activities such as 'morning sharing', or a coffee and chat break. Usually after this time, fatigue sets in and focus is lost.

Preparation

Time: 15 minutes prior to starting time

- ◉ Set up a circle of chairs, leaving spaces for wheelchairs if necessary.
- ◉ Play calming music as participants enter the program space.

Welcome

Time: 5 minutes

Aim

To greet and orient participants.

Description

Welcome everyone to the dance/movement program, offer assistance to get seated and explain the plan for the session. Greet each person individually within the group and encourage a response. A rhythmic song is a fun way of doing this (see Chapter 2, page 30).

Warm-up

Time: 10 minutes

Choose one of these activities

Chair warm-up

Aim

This section provides a warm-up for the whole body, beginning at the bottom (i.e. feet), using simple movements to bring awareness to each body part.

Description

Some suitable movements include:

- *feet:* Heel and toe lifts, circling ankles, turning toes inward and outward, curling and then lifting the toes.
- *knees and legs:* Walking in place, lifting knees, moving knees together and apart.
- *shoulders:* Lifting and releasing shoulders, circling them forwards and backwards.
- *arms and hands:* Reaching arms forward, upward, out to the sides and down at the sides, arm circles and sweeps, elbow and wrists bends, opening and closing hands and fingers (such as moving the fingers apart and together or simulated piano playing).
- *trunk:* Rocking the whole body forwards and backwards, twisting to right and left side, tilting the body to the right and left side.
- *head:* Slow, gentle head turns, head drops, chin lifts.
  (Adapted from Clark 1998.)

Music

Something lively but not too fast.

- Tom Jones, (1992), *Greatest Hits of Tom Jones.*
- Elton John, (1990), *The Very Best of Elton John.*

Balloon game

Aim

To develop focus and interaction with others.

Description

Begin by batting a balloon from one member to another. Participants can be encouraged to make eye contact with the person they have chosen to receive the balloon, or make a sound to alert the prospective recipient. People with speech can be encouraged to say the name of the person they are directing the balloon to. Balloons are ideal for this kind of activity as their lightness enables even the weakest movement to have an obvious impact. Their sustained speed allows for slow responses. They are also unlikely to cause any injury, even if the receiver misses their catch.

Variations

- ◎ 'Keep it up' game. Count how many times the balloon can be hit before it touches the floor. Try to improve on the record each time.
- ◎ Add extra balloon/s to encourage slightly speedier reactions and a livelier game.
- ◎ Specify a response. Some ideas for this include:
  - catch the balloon and carry it to a someone else.
  - hit it with a particular body part, e.g. head, elbow, forearm, nose.
  - don't leave your seat to touch it.

Music

Music with a steady buoyant rhythm that envigorates, such as:

- ◎ New Flamenco (1999), *Gypsy Soul*.
- ◎ Various artists (1995), *Café del Mar*, Vol. 2, Track 6.

Stretch and strengthen

Time: 10 minutes

Pursed lips breathing

A breathing exercise is a good starting point for stretches. Rimmer's (1998) pursed lips breathing exercise increases the amount of air taken into the lungs.

- ◎ Inhale slowly through the nose, keeping the mouth closed
- ◎ Pucker the lips as if trying to whistle.
- ◎ Exhale slowly, blowing the air through pursed lips.
- ◎ Exhalation should be as least twice as long as inhalation. Begin with a two-second inhalation and a four-second exhalation.
- ◎ Rest and repeat several times.

Stretches

Each activity should be performed using both sides of the body.

- ◎ *Ear-to-shoulder stretches*: Lower ear to shoulder, then return to centre.
- ◎ *Neck rotation:* Turn head to shoulder.
- ◎ *Shoulder circle:* Circle the shoulders, forward, up, backwards and down. Reverse.
- ◎ *Spine extensions:* Place hands on thighs, then gently round and extend the back.
- ◎ *Arm lifts:* Lift and curve arms overhead, as if holding a big round ball above the head.

- ◎ *Stretch the trunk:* Turn torso to the side, holding the same side of the chair with both hands.
- ◎ *Stretch the chest and shoulders:* Bend both arms at the elbow and cross them behind the back.
- ◎ *Hamstring stretch:* Place heel on floor in front of the body and pull toes towards you, gradually bending forward at the hips.
- ◎ *Stretch inner thighs:* Separate knees as far as possible.
- ◎ *Stretch outer thighs:* Cross one leg over the other.
- ◎ *Stretch shin and calves:* Flex and point toes.

Music

Something lyrical and flowing, with some energy and strength like:

- ◎ Louis Armstrong, 'What a Wonderful World'
- ◎ Billie Holiday (1990), *Best of Billie Holiday*.

Seated stretch with scarves

This activity, described in Chapter 2 (page 56), is ideal for older adults, especially those who might be inspired by the added motivation of a colourful prop.

Social dance

Time: 10 minutes

Aim

After the slower pace of the stretch, participants may have recovered enough to go back into a lively activity. This is often people's favourite part of the session, when they feel that they are really 'dancing'.

Description

The dance can be something that members are already familiar with, such as a social dance like 'The Hokey Pokey', 'The Pride of Erin', 'The Barn Dance' or rock 'n' roll. It can also be something new that is built up from earlier class activities.

To extend participants' stamina in this section, opportunities to observe others can be provided. This will allow those who need a rest to take it, without the whole class having to come to a standstill. The leader might ask one couple who have come up with an interesting idea or who are working well together to demonstrate one section of the dance to the rest of the group.

The example below describes how a performance item developed out of movements from a seated warm-up. The feeling of fun that it inspired led the group into creation of a performance masterpiece! So much energy was generated, in fact, that many members ended up getting right out of the chairs, and the dance became only nominally a chair dance.

Hill Billy Cajun Stamping Dance

Participants had been enjoying a very lively warm-up to some Cajun country music. This music gave the activity a bouncy and fun dynamic. Clapping and stamping happened almost involuntarily, and with that came loud and joyful vocalisations. ('Yee ha' was modelled by me (Kim) first!) I then led the group into experimentation with body percussion movements, including slapping of knees, thighs and imaginary long boots, pitter-patter with fingers on their heads, beating of chests, etc. The dance went like this:

◎ Participants sit on chairs in a row facing the audience.

◎ *Feet begin to move:* Toes move up and down, heels up and down, toes and heels up and down, toes move out and in, heels out and in.

◎ Knees open and close, hands are placed on knees crossing over with movement of the knees.

◎ *Interaction:* Performers reach out to tap their neighbour's knees.

◎ Clap a 'High 5' with a neighbour.

◎ Standing solos: e.g. one person walks to the front of the row of seated dancers, then walks along the row clapping hands with each person as they pass. Or they begin by walking to the back of the row, then walk along the row tapping the shoulders of each person as they pass.

◎ *Bum slap:* Turn back to audience and slap your bottom.

◎ All members travel (walk, skip, gallop) around chairs to change position, like a game of '*musical chairs*'.

◎ *Say goodbye:* Each dancer creates an individual way to finish the dance, e.g. blowing a kiss, taking a bow or curtseying, or repeating a favourite movement made earlier to create a kind of movement signature.

Music
Various artists, (2001) *Absolutely the Best of Cajun and Zydeco.*

Relaxation

Time: 10 minutes

Seated relaxation activities like 'Head, neck and shoulder massage' or 'Spine stretch', described in Chapter 2, are ideal for this age group.

Working with high-support needs participants

What are high support needs?

People who need assistance to facilitate their participation in a program can be considered to have high support needs. This may be due to physical disabilities that restrict mobility, sight and/or hearing. There are also people who have a need for one-to-one support because of behavioural challenges and/or emotional distress they experience in a group situation. The level of support needed by a person does not necessarily correspond with the severity of their disability. Some people have 'acquired' their level of disability through institutionalisation and a deficit of meaningful, caring and ongoing human relationships. Often what 'high support' people have in common is a coping strategy of shutting down from the outside world, building a highly individualised expression of self and means of communication based on sounds, gestures and postures. This group can be the most challenging, not only because of their disabilities but because of their physical limits. Their bodies can often be stuck in heavy weight, with little or no flow or dynamic range and extreme awkwardness.

The challenge and delight of working with such people is to step into their world and ignite the spark of human relationship that can lead to meaningful communication. Valuing the uniqueness of each person's body, movement (no matter how restricted) and personal space immediately creates a motivation for working towards engagement with the most disconnected individual. If approached from this angle and with these values, dance is possible with anyone.

Expectations

When planning and facilitating sessions for people with high support needs it is important to be flexible in what you expect to achieve. At one of the centres where I (Jenny) work, it took two months of weekly sessions before most of the group would sit in a circle for the start of the session. Even after this time some members still preferred the safety of a corner. With a high-support needs group, the basic structure and skills needed for participating in a dance programs, for example, forming a circle, moving and stopping and co-operating with a partner, cannot be taken as an essential starting point. Rather, they are to be worked towards over a period of time. The most important expectation to have is that the group leader is willing to engage with group members through music and movement and that she or he values and encourages the slightest offer of movement made by participants. It is helpful to let go of expectations and simply believe in the innate capacity of the body/human spirit to move and find an expression through dance, whatever that dance may be.

Attunement

Instead of planning movements or dances for the session, it might be necessary to work with any movement response offered by the participants. This may be a handshake, a smile, an eye-blink, rocking, jumping, reaching, retreating or standing still. Any movement offered by a participant can be responded to by the group leader, who can mirror, contrast, amplify, reduce and use points of contact and stillness. An explanation of these movement responses are listed:

◎ *Mirror:* This is reflecting back to the mover their own movement as if they are looking in a mirror. This can be done standing side to side or face to face with a person.

◎ *Amplify:* The same as mirroring, except that the group leader/support worker makes their movement bigger in response.

◎ *Reduce:* Again the same as mirroring, except that the group leader/support worker makes their movement smaller in response.

◎ *Contrast:* This is responding with a movement that expresses the opposite of what the mover is doing. For example, a small movement of a participant's hand could be contrasted by a small movement of the leader's leg.

◎ *Points of contact:* Finding parts of a person's body on which to rest, for example, back to back or leaning on a shoulder. Finding parts of a person's body to touch such as a hand, elbow or knee. When approached in this way, a dance can be created with someone if they are willing, even if they are standing still.

◎ *Stillness:* Enjoy moments of stillness by standing, sitting or lying still next to someone.

By responding to participants' movements with attention to detail, sensitivity and playfulness, movement communication will open up. The group leader needs to be tuned in and ready to respond to anything that may emerge. Being flexible, however, does not mean working with the absence of structure. For the development of trust and for the potential growth of group interaction, it is important that a session has a clear beginning, middle and end.

Group leader provides the connection

When working with high-support needs participants, the group leader has the challenging role of facilitating a group process while focusing on individuals in the group in a one-to-one relationship. This requires the ability to step from one individual to another while maintaining a link with the group as a whole. The group leader dancing between the members of the group, and weaving a connection, may be the only connection present if group members have retreated into their own world. This is the experience I (Jenny) have had when working with people who have been institutionalised from an early age.

The group leader needs to be able to move from this one-to-one engagement into linking other group members through dance. This requires the group leader to develop an awareness of when an individual may be ready to connect with others. This may simply mean knowing when to offer a hand so that a dance between two people becomes a dance between three. When working with these participants, it can be a great joy when the social dimension emerges and the circle that is desired appears.

Dance therapy versus creative dance

A dance therapy process is more appropriate than educational- or performance-focused creative dance for people with high support needs. For these clients, the primary aim is to establish trusting relationships through the use of movement and the body. Secondary aims would be the development of expression through movement, playfulness and experience of different rhythms and variations in mood. While a creative dance program would also value building relationships, it also aims to extend movement through a range of movement experiences. The opportunity to perform work either in front of the group or to an invited audience is a skill developed in creative movement classes that would not be appropriate in a group of participants with high support needs.

A group leader running a dance program for people with high support needs must understand the limitations in terms of exploring movement and feel excited about the potential for engagement with people who are amongst the most marginalised members of our community.

Staffing issue: Support workers and shared outcomes

When working with participants who have high support needs, an ideal ratio is two participants to one support worker. In practice, however, this ratio will often vary, depending upon the availability of funding and staff. A leader should never attempt to run a group of three or more high-support needs participants on their own, as it will be difficult to meet clients' needs and injury may occur. When working with support staff it is important to communicate to them the intention of the program and strategies for how to achieve outcomes, so that they can assist in the most supportive way possible. For example, achieving a level of attunement with participants would be a more desirable outcome than aiming for a vigorous physical workout that may require coercion. This may be a challenge for some support workers who have a preconceived idea or experience of dance sessions being the time when everyone 'gets up to boogie'.

Support workers can be a great asset, not only for hands-on assistance, but also for the history and understanding of their clients that they can bring. They are likely to be able to provide information on how to deal with particular behaviours and, most importantly, the likes and dislikes of their clients. A group of high-support needs participants will function better if there is a friendly and supportive relationship between the group leader and support workers.

The group leader may at times need to be flexible in order to incorporate the personality and gifts of a worker. I (Jenny) have had the great pleasure of working at different centres with talented musicians who are employed as carers. These people have helped bring life and energy to dance sessions with their music, by playing instruments such as piano, guitar or drums.

However, not all support staff will engage in a dance program with enthusiasm. To encourage an unengaged support worker to feel more part of the program the leader might ask for their ideas and suggest they bring some of their favourite music to the session. A support worker who is not willing to participate with enthusiasm can be more inhibiting than helpful to a program. If a group leader has no success with these suggested strategies, the problem will need to be discussed with that staff member first, and then if no solution is reached, with their manager.

Toiletting and physical care

Participants may need to be toiletted during the program. This obviously must be a priority, but can be frustrating when the group or the individual is in the middle of an activity. The leader must be willing to let go of what they are doing in order to accommodate such needs and to look for ways to move on with the program. A specialist group leader working in a centre is usually exempt from helping with toiletting. This is to protect the client's privacy and also so that they are assisted in the most professional way. It is important for the comfort and safety of all that these roles and responsibilities are clarified.

Wanderers

Some participants, especially people with autism, may find it difficult to stay in the room for an extended length of time. This may mean that support workers will be absent while they spend some time-out with a group member or search for someone who has wandered off. Occasionally a group leader may need to abandon a program to assist with locating or placating a participant.

Lifting

There is usually some manual lifting involved with high-support needs participants. Support workers will have the training to deal with this and will generally be the ones to do most of the lifting and transfers. However, a group leader is likely to have to give physical support to assist participants to dance, so some training in lifting techniques is advisable, as is the sense to work safely within one's own lifting capabilities.

Sample lesson for high-support needs participants

The lesson detailed below is based on a 60-minute session with eight participants and two support workers. This is a good time frame to begin with as it does not over-stretch participants' concentration or the length of time spent in one room. As the program develops and participants' likes and dislikes become known, adjustments can be made. Within six months, it is reasonable to expect that the session could extend to 75 minutes by extending the 'free dance' section and relaxation time. In most cases the maximum desirable length of a session is 90 minutes. Usually after this time fatigue sets in and focus is lost.

It would be unrealistic to run a session for high support people with more than 10 participants because the nature of the work is primarily one-to-one. To run a successful program, the ideal ratio would be three support workers and a group leader with 10 participants.

This 60-minute session would also be suitable for a small group of four participants and one support worker. With a small group, it is less of a challenge to maintain focus and engagement, so a 60-minute session can be just right for a concentrated effort from staff and participants.

Preparation

Time: 15 minutes prior to starting time.

- ◉   Set up a circle of chairs, leaving spaces for wheelchairs if necessary.
- ◉   Play calming music as participants enter program space.

Welcome

Time: 10 minutes

Hello game or song

Aim
To greet and orientate participants.

Description
Greet each person individually within the group. Wait for each person's response (a wave, smile, eye contact, vocalisation, beat a drum). A rhythmic song is a fun way of doing this, such as those described in Chapter 2, page 30.

Focus exercise

Aim
To settle the group and bring attention to the present moment, so that all group members are ready for participation in the dance session.

Description
Passing a big balloon (light weight) or bean bag (strong weight)

The group leader stands in the centre and passes a bag or balloon to a participant and encourages the participant to pass it back to the leader. The leader continues around the circle, passing the bag to each person and saying their name. This is a good opportunity to give some encouraging feedback, for example, 'Guy, fantastic throw' or 'Good catching Sonny'.

or

Pass the balloon/bean bag around the circle clockwise and then anti-clockwise.

Music
Calm and inspiring music like *Amelie Soundtrack*, Track 4.

Warm-up

Time: 10 minutes

Kicking with exercise ball

Aim
To begin physical engagement and establish connection between group members, heighten awareness of self and others.

Description

Participants kick the ball to another member across the circle. They can be encouraged to make eye contact, smile or point to the person to whom they are directing the ball before kicking. Participants who are unable to move their legs independently will need assistance (co-active participation).

Music

Playful:

◎   Bert Kaempfert, *Roses*, tracks 10–12

◎   Café del Mar, *Ibiza*.

Sensory work with ribbons

Aim

Using a tactile prop to stimulate engagement, encourage flow quality and emotion.

Description

Collection of different textured ribbons or fabric (e.g. smooth, furry, coarse) are needed for this exercise. The group leader and support staff work one-on-one for about two to three minutes with each person around the circle. Participants are encouraged to reach for, touch and manipulate the ribbons, while the leader looks for ways to extend movements such as rocking back and forward as the participant and leader hold opposite ends of the ribbon. A game of tug-of-war can be fun when, instead of rocking back and forwards, each person pulls the ribbon in their own direction.

Music

Music to encourage flow quality in movement:

◎   Gypsy Soul (1998) *New Flamenco, Narada*, includes flowing tracks, especially track 2.

Group dance

Time: 10 minutes

Social dance

Aim

Engaging individuals and establishing connection between group members using well known tunes and adapting basic folk dances.

Description: '*Hokey Pokey*'

For people who cannot initiate their own movement, this can be done with co-active facilitation while seated on a chair or in a wheelchair. An activity like this is suitable for people who are non-ambulant and make little self-initiated movement. This activity provides a good opportunity for establishing eye contact with participants in a playful way.

Group members sit in a circle. The group leader and support workers form an inside circle, and stand in front of a participant. When the song says:

◎   '*Put your right arm in*': Support worker holds or touches right hand of participant.

◎ *'Put your right hand out'*: Support worker lets go of participant's hand.

◎ *'Put your right hand in'*: Repeat previous step

◎ *'And shake it all about'*: Support worker and participant shake hands.

◎ *'You do the Hokey Pokey'*: Support worker places hands on knees of participants and firmly but gently rocks the knees from side to side.

◎ *'And you turn around'*: Support worker circles the seated participant, keeping eye contact.

◎ *'And that's what it's all about'*: Support worker and participant clap hands.

◎ *'Oh, the Hokey Pokey, Oh, the Hokey Pokey'*: Support worker moves in towards participant to clap a *'Hi 5'* with both hands. If this is not possible for the participant, the support worker raises his or her hands above his or her head and then gently brings them down to touch the participant's shoulders and knees.

◎ *'And that's what it's all about'*: Clap hands together

◎ Support worker moves around the circle to the right and begins again with the next group member.

or

Description: *'Chicken Dance' (or 'Little Bird Dance')*
The *'Chicken Dance'* is made up of movements of the shoulders, hips and hands. For people who have restricted movement, these body parts can be brought into awareness through touch and stimulated through gentle, slow movement. Adapting the *'Chicken Dance'*, with its familiar and lively music, is a fun way to turn movement into a dance.

◎ Participants sit in a circle. The group leader and assistant/s stand face to face with a partner standing/sitting inside the circle. Partners greet each other with a smile.

◎ *'A little bit of this'*: Leader firmly but gently places hands on partner's shoulders, slowly rocking them side to side while singing along with the song.

◎ *'And a little bit of that'*: Leader move to their partner's hips and place hands firmly but gently on the hips, repeat rocking motion and singing along with them.

◎ *'And shake your hands'*: Leader then places his/her hands together with partner's hand (possible handholds include palm to palm, handshake, cupping both hands around partner's hands), repeating rocking motion and sings along.

◎ *'Around and round in circles'*: Group leader and assistant/s stand up and weave around the circle of seated participants, moving in front of and behind them, touching each person on the shoulder or briefly holding their hand as they pass.

When the chorus is finished, the leader stands in front of a new partner ready to begin again.

Music
Master Sounds (1998) *The Bird Dance and Other Party Dance Favourites*, includes 'The Chicken Dance' ('The Bird Dance') and 'The Hokey Pokey'.

Free dance

Time: 15 minutes

Creative dance

Aim

Independent or assisted self-expression through movement.

Description

This is an opportunity for participants to move around the room independently, with assistance or in their wheelchair, as appropriate. Begin by moving all the chairs to the side of the room to create a clear space. Play participants' favourite music, taking turns week by week so that everyone has a chance to share their choices. Sometimes the group leader may wish to choose a style of music to help develop particular movement quality.

If there is not much spontaneous or free-flow movement happening use the techniques described at the beginning of this section under 'Attunement' (page 101).

The following music recordings can be helpful to inspire participants to move and dance.

Music

Offer a variety of rhythms, styles and era:

- Mickey Hart (1991), *Planet Drum*, African drumming
- Tribal Trance (1998), *Minjahra*, strong rhythms and melodic vocals
- Hot Toddy (1999), *Celtic Fire*, fun energetic Celtic
- New Flamenco (1998), *Gypsy Soul*, rhythmic, energetic and flowing
- *Afro Latino* (1998), rhythmic and joyful.

Relaxation

Time: 10 minutes

Aim

To release tension from body and mind.

Description

The group returns to the circle, as for the beginning of the session. The group leader and support workers offer each group member a shoulder massage and an arm stretch. Some participants may not enjoy physical contact or may be uncomfortable with a person standing behind them. An alternative strategy is the use of soft brushes (shaving brushes or make-up brushes) to gently stroke body parts such as palms, fingers, neck and face, depending on what seems to be most relaxing for the participant. Another possibility is to use a piece of soft fabric and move it towards and away from the participant in a wave-like motion so that the fabric gently touches and retreats from their face.

or

If there is enough time and sufficient support staff for lifting, participants may enjoy relaxation time by lying in a beanbag rather than sitting up in their chair. Hand and foot massage are very enjoyable from this position. It could also be time to simply sit and listen to a piece of beautiful music.

Music

Calm and soothing

◉ ABC Classics (1998) *The Swoon Collection I, II & II,*

◉ Jan Garbarek/the Hillard Ensemble (1994) *Officium,*

◉ Beethoven, 'Pastoral Symphony Awakening of Joyful Feelings'.

Goodbye

Time: 5 minutes

Say goodbye to each person and acknowledge their contribution to the session. For example, 'Rose, it was exciting to see you kick the ball across the room today'. Discover the way each participant can initiate a goodbye, for example, with a wave, a handshake or a smile, and encourage this as their personal way of saying goodbye.

Chapter 5

Extending the creative dance medium

There are a number of ways to extend the experience of learning through creative dance, including the use of props, other dance styles such as folk and social dance and the incorporation of art forms such as drama, music, poetry and film. In this chapter we look at some of the ways in which they can be used to enrich dance programs for people with intellectual disabilities.

Working with props

Props can be used to enhance participants' involvement in a creative dance process by creating new and stimulating visual and sensory experiences. They can be useful for motivating those who have trouble connecting with others, as props can provide a non-threatening link. People with autism, for example, are often more comfortable interacting with objects than with people, so an indirect link with others in the group via a prop may be more manageable. Props can also help to focus the attention of those who have difficulty concentrating.

Balls

Using balls to create connection
Balls can help create a point of connection, especially for people with high support needs. Activities such as passing the ball backwards and forwards between leader and members can prompt participants to reach in all directions to catch it. Passing and catching also encourage eye focus, hand–eye co-ordination and full arm extension. Hand-sized balls are the easiest to manage for people with restricted movement.

Providing sensory stimulation
Different textured balls are excellent for sensory stimulation for hands and fingers. Textures can include smooth, bubbly, rubbery and coarse. Balls of different weight can add another dimension.

A ball as a facilitating device
A ball can be a good tool for facilitating a group discussion. As a ball is passed around the group, the person holding it is given the opportunity to speak uninterrupted. The ball can create a clear focus for the group and give authority to the person holding it. Once the person holding the ball has finished sharing their ideas they can pass the ball to a person of their choice in the group. This is helpful in overcoming the problem of simultaneous conversations in a noisy group, and as a means of encouraging quieter members to contribute to a group

discussion. It also adds an element of surprise that will keep members focused. It is a good idea to have a special ball just for this activity so that it works as a cue for silence and focus. Choose one that is clearly visible in size and colour.

Various activities with small, medium and large physio balls

Buoyant soft plastic 'physio' balls offer a range of possibilities for energetic and relaxing activities.

- ◉ *Small*: Throwing a small physio ball is a good activity for a group of varying abilities, especially people with independent skills. Lifting the ball and directing it carefully to another member requires upper body strength and judgment. This activity is best suited to a dance venue that has a lot of space and high windows, such as a gymnasium, or it could be done outside on a nice day.

- ◉ *Medium:* Kicking a medium-sized physio ball is a good activity for people with high support needs. Position the group into a close circle so that participants are able to clearly focus on people sitting on the opposite side. The object is to choose another person in the circle and kick the ball to them. To begin, the ball should be placed at the feet of the member who volunteers to go first. If participants can use verbal language they can say the name of the person to whom they are directing the ball as they kick. If they don't have language skills they can make eye contact with that person. As the group becomes more skilled at kicking, the circle can become wider to encourage larger and stronger movements.

- ◉ *Large:* Relaxing over a large physio ball can be a pleasurable experience for people with all levels of disability. Participants lie over the ball so that their body forms a C shape, with chest, abdomen and arms falling over the curve of the ball. The group leader can gently rock the ball as a way of encouraging relaxation. This activity can be helpful to people who have high body tone, as the total support provided by the ball encourages the release of tension. Do not persist with this activity, however, if a participant is unwilling or if it triggers tonal patterns that increase body tension. This will be evident if the body of the person on the ball becomes rigid.

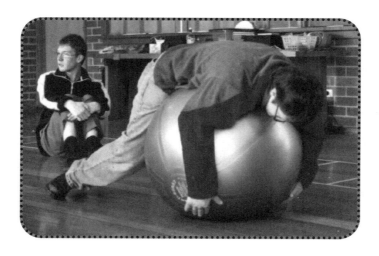

Where to get balls

Small balls can be purchased from toy shops, reject shops, sports stores and opportunity shops. Physio balls can be purchased from physiotherapy suppliers, gymnasiums and sports stores.

Bubble wrap

This is a creative way of articulating movement through fingers, hands, feet and toes and at the same time making a 'bubble popping' soundscape*.

Activities for hands

◎ Each participant holds a small square of bubble wrap (approximately 30 cm x 30 cm).

◎ Using hands and fingers, participants twist the bubble wrap to make the bubbles pop. This will be an enjoyable challenge for people who find it difficult to access strength in movement.

◎ Create a soundscape by popping bubbles. One person at a time around the circle can make their bubbles 'pop and crackle', while the rest of the group listens. Continue with each person following quickly after the other, aiming for no quiet gaps in between.

Activities for feet

◎ Make a 'catwalk' down the length of the dance space with bubble wrap. Secure bubble wrap to the floor with masking tape.

◎ Heighten the sensory experience and increase full foot articulation by taking shoes off.

◎ Participants walk down the length of the bubble wrap one by one with the intention of squashing the bubbles. Like the hand exercise, this will be an enjoyable challenge for those people who find accessing strength difficult.

◎ Participants can be encouraged to use different parts of their feet to squash the bubbles, e.g. big and little toes, heels, balls, outside and inside of the feet.

Where to get bubble wrap

Bubble wrap can be purchased by the metre from stationery suppliers.

Simon uses his feet to pop all the bubbles

Simon is a BreakOut member who often needs a lot of prompting to engage physically in any activity. Due to his autism, Simon is often disconnected from the group and happily dreaming in his own world. To our surprise, we found the bubble wrap activity fully engaged Simon's attention and physical skills. When it was his turn to walk down the 'catwalk', he applied all his concentration to popping as many bubbles as he could, using all the parts of his feet. Simon found all of these foot-parts without a single word of prompting. While this activity brought out his autistic tendency to focus on detail, Simon was the only group member able to articulate every part of his feet successfully. He finished the activity with a look of contentment on his face.

*This idea originally came from Joy, (2000)

Candles
Creating magic, developing focus, exploring space

Tea candles placed around the dance space can create a magical environment, especially if the lights are turned out. Members can be invited to find their own pathway around and through the candles. A performance space set up in this way can encourage those people who have a preference for staying within the safety of their own personal space to move out of it and explore the space in the room.

Where to get tea candles
Tea candles can be purchased very cheaply from supermarkets and variety stores.

Candles help create focus and transformation

I (Kim) used candles with great success to create focus in a dance/drama class with a group of mildly intellectually disabled teenagers. This group's learning was being seriously challenged by students' lack of focus and constant lapses into unhelpful behaviours such as name-calling and teasing. I decided that the creation of a super-ordinary environment might move these young people out of the mundane and into the transformative magic of performance.

Before the students arrived, I closed the curtains, turned off the lights in the dance space and lit tea candles placed all over the floor. I met the students in the foyer and set the scene for magic by asking them all to take off their shoes, coats and bags before they entered. Then, unencumbered by objects from the everyday world, we quietly did a breathing activity together to bring their focus inward. Once quiet and focus was established, I turned on some very meditative music, silently opened one small door into the space and asked them to silently (no voice, no body sounds) move through and around the candles.

Then, once I had established that they could co-operate and manipulate themselves safely through this slightly dangerous environment, I asked the students to pick up the candles and move without letting the candle blow out. This required very slow, careful and focused movements, and proved quite a challenge.

The rest of the session went much better that day, as students had been moved from their everyday patterns of movement and relationship into a quieter, more focused state of being. We continued to use the candle dance as a 'warm-up' activity, the reverse of a more normal pattern of a physically demanding and energy increasing warm-up. Gradually over ten weeks, we did manage to create two pieces for an end-of-term performance, one of them a choreography of the candle dance. The event was spellbinding, and seemed to create the same magic for the audience as it had for the performers.

Music
The music I used was 'China on a Bicycle' by Southern Crossings on their self-titled album, but other music that has a meditative quality, such as Tibetan meditation or Gregorian chants, would also be suitable.

Cloaks

A floor-length velvet cloak can stimulate interesting movement experiences and be useful for developing a sense of sustainment, focus and bound flow. The weight and length of the cloak has the effect of slowing down and restricting movement. This can be useful for those who have trouble focusing attention, or accessing qualities of sustainment in movement, like people with ADHD. An elegant costume like this cloak can also help create a sense of magical transformation and easier access to a different character.

Where to get cloaks
Try opportunity shops or costume hire shops. Makeshift cloaks can be made from lengths of velvet fastened around dancers' necks.

Cloaks and stirring music create sense of majesty and dignity

At the first of BreakOut's performances that I (Kim) ever saw, I watched members of the older adult group perform a very moving processional dance accompanied by a stirring Gregorian chant. The sense of dignity and clear focus created by this slow and gracious procession was intensified by the dancers' costumes of long velvet cloaks. This dance seemed a very ennobling event and one that confirmed my view of the value of dance, even for these not-so-young performers.

Fabrics

Making waves with chiffon

One long piece of chiffon (approximately 10 m x 1 m) is used to shape, direct and extend movement.

Aim
To develop movement at high level, full body stretch, articulation of hands and fingers, spinal mobility.

Description
The fabric is held and manipulated by two people, along the length of the dance space. The people holding the fabric stretch it out wide and long between them, while participants move under, around, over and through it. Changing the level of the fabric will encourage participants to change the level of their movements.

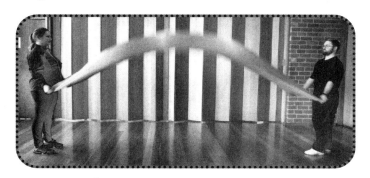

◎ As participants travel under the fabric, they stretch up as if they are reaching for the sky. If the fabric is held low, participants have to bend low to get under it.

◎ If the fabric is floated up and down like a wave, participants can travel under it without letting it touch their bodies (developing speed, agility, body awareness), or try and allow it to touch certain body parts e.g., only head, right shoulder, elbow or forearm (developing body awareness, articulation, co-ordination, motor planning).

◎ Participants can experiment with different ways of travelling under it. The leader can use moving words like *spinning, rolling, reaching, back first* to stimulate ideas.

Working together two people find a way to move together through the waves. The two might:

- start at the same end of the fabric, moving together, in canon or unsynchronised
- start at opposite ends of the fabric, moving together, in canon or unsynchronised
- move on opposite sides of the fabric, e.g. one goes over while the other goes under (developing creativity, co-operation, co-ordination).

Fabric is manipulated by two people, one who is stationary and one who moves

Aim
To develop co-ordination, co-operation

Description
Solo/small group 'winding'. The mover might 'wind' him/herself in and out of fabric, either alone, or including others.

Variation
The group is connected by the fabric.

Aim
For the mover to develop leadership, movement creativity, co-ordination; for group members to develop focus, connection, co-operation, co-ordination.

Description
The 'mover' finds a way to connect all the people in the room with the fabric. They might be just touching the fabric with their hands or another body part, or they might be wrapped in it. The activity might finish with the whole group in the connected position, or they might attempt to move together, keeping the connection with each other through the fabric.

Fabric manipulated by two people who are moving

Aim
To develop the use of directions in space, changes in level of movement, engagement, relationship, co-ordination.

◎ *Partner work:* The two dancers hold opposite ends of the fabric and travel through the space, experimenting with movement directions such as towards and away from each other, over and under, tangle/untangle.

Variation

◎　*Whole group activity:* Using the fabric each group member finds their own way to join in and become part of a group sculpture. This could be a static pose or part of a flowing group movement.

Music

To create a dreamy atmosphere that allows for large, flowing, sustained movements:

◎　Enya (1997), *Paint the Sky with Stars*, tracks 8, 12, 13

◎　Handel's 'Water Music', or

◎　*Best of Romantic Piano Music* (1994)

◎　To create focus on connectedness with others, use a more lively piece like 'Song Sung Blue' by Neil Diamond. This will create a fun atmosphere, while still allowing for flow quality. A familiar tune will often inspire participants to sing along.

◎　To create dramatic, strong, energetic movements, stormy music like Vaughan Williams' (1995) *A Sea Symphony*

◎　Bach, *Brandenburg Concerto No. 3 – Allegro*.

Fabric wall 'finish line'

Aim

To encourage fast speed, direction, focus, energy.

Description

Use a large piece of lycra held across the dance space to create a safe and motivating finish line. Participants run headlong into the fabric for a soft landing.

Fabric wall shapes and shadows

Aim

To develop body awareness and articulation, choice and decision making, creative thinking.

Description

Participants take turns to stand behind the fabric and press body parts against it to make shapes visible to the rest of the group.

The fabric wall gets people talking

In one of my (Jenny's) groups of adults with mild intellectual disabilities, this activity of making shapes from behind a piece of fabric provoked a very lively discussion about group members' interest in films, especially those of the horror genre. This topic led on to a lively discussion about ghosts and other-worldly experiences. I had never heard class members talk so much or so animatedly! This experience helped me get to know participants' lives and interests in a way I never had before, despite meeting them in dance class weekly for two years. We followed the talking with related movement experiences, and finished up having one of the most enjoyable and stimulating sessions ever.

Fans and water

Hot weather activities using fans, water and fresh mint

Props

- ◎ Large bowl filled with cool water, and floating, fresh mint leaves
- ◎ Set of one-person sized fans
- ◎ Two giant rush fans.

Aim

In very hot weather, it is important to provide activities that do not add to participants' discomfort, especially those older adults who have difficulty with stamina and balance. The following activities were created for a group of older adults on a very hot morning. Some activities involved movement around the space, but many were done seated to reduce exertion.

'Warm-up' (really cool-down on this occasion!)

Aim

Body awareness, naming and focusing on body parts.

Description

Fanning: Participants take a fan each and begin by fanning body parts in succession, especially the parts that are likely to be hot and sticky, including scalp, forehead, ears, under the chin, armpits, back of neck, elbow creases, palms, sides of torso, waist, thighs, under knee, ankles, under feet, toes.

Stretching with water

Description

Participants dip hands into the bowl, then with wet fingers, stretch to touch body parts, for example:

- ◎ fingertips reach up and behind the neck
- ◎ hands stretch towards knees and then toes
- ◎ palms of hands reach to soles of feet (crossing right hand to left foot and vice-versa)
- ◎ both hands touch together behind the back
- ◎ both hands touch together under the knees
- ◎ right hand reaches to left side of the waist, then reverse movement.

Improvised fan dance

Description

- ◎ *Preparation:* Sitting in a circle, participants hold their fans and experiment with movements and movement qualities. Leader and any verbal participants can suggest words that relate to the movements the group are making: for example, floating, fluttering, swooping, spinning, twirling. Participants can experiment with movements that match those words.

- *Create a circle:* All members face inwards and hold fans together in the centre of a tight circle.

- *Fans move together:* All fans move together on the spot with perhaps a small flutter.

- *Up and down, out and in:* All fans move up and down together; in and out together, with participants still standing (or sitting) facing each other in a circle.

- *Solos:* One member at a time lifts their fan up and out of the circle, and creates his/her own movements for a few moments, before coming back to the centre circle.

- *Taking off:* All members, led by their fans, fly up and out of the circle and out into the rest of the space. Each person creates their own shapes, and movements as they travel.

- *Partner work:* Participants move towards a partner. Face to face, the two find a way to move together with their fans, perhaps touching; moving towards and away from each other, over and under, together and in canon.

- *Group together:* Back to back circle; all dancers come together to create a circle, this time standing or sitting with backs together: fans fluttering up and down in canon to create a wave-like motion.

- *Finale:* Fans flutter up for one last time, then slowly down and stop. Dancers slowly turn towards centre of circle, lifting fans up, over and down.

Music
Something flowing, relaxed and watery such as:
- Mozart, 'Come Sweet May'
- Handel, 'Water Music'
- Howlin Wind (1995), *Dugong Lullaby*, especially Tracks 1, 8 and 9.

Relaxation with giant fan

Description
Participants sit or lie in constructive rest position. Using giant fans, staff members gently fan over the group, allowing the moving air to create a sense of cool and restfulness.

Alternative
The 'Flying Wave' relaxation, as described in Chapter 2 (page 59). Suitable only for class members who can lie on the floor.

Music
- Howlin Wind (1995), *Dugong Lullaby*, especially Tracks 2, 6 and 10
- James Galway, *Songs of the Seashore*.

Where to get giant fans
Asian grocery or variety store, haberdashery shops, opportunity shops.

Giant elastic

Aim

A giant elastic can be very useful for facilitating group co-operation and connection, especially in the early stages when a group is learning to make a circle and experiment with concepts of shape, such as expanding and contracting. Note that it does require participants to have enough both strength and flexibility in their hands to be able to hold the elastic.

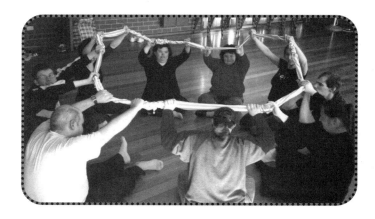

Description

Begin activities with the elastic while the group is seated on the floor or chairs to avoid spontaneous experimentation that could put people with balance problems at risk. The elastic is an excellent means of extending the range of movement for a group with mixed abilities and older adults.

The group sits on chairs in a circle, holding the elastic with their hands. Begin by moving with the elastic at a slow to moderate pace to accommodate all members. Movements to try can include:

- rocking from side to side
- rocking forwards and extending the elastic into the middle of the circle
- rocking backwards, pulling elastic back onto the chest. Repeat in a sequence moving forward and backwards
- extending elastic down to touch toes
- extending elastic high to touch the ceiling.

At a faster pace, try:

- releasing one hand at a time from the elastic
- extending the released arm high into the air.

How to make a giant elastic

You will need a piece of elastic approximately 5 m long x 8 cm wide.

- Join the elastic so that it makes a circle, stitching the ends firmly together (preferably by sewing machine, for added strength).

◉ Use a stretch knit fabric or fabric cut on the bias to make a cover for the elastic. Make the cover 1 1/2 times as large as the elastic so that it can stretch far enough. Plain fabric is preferable to reduce the possibility of people with autism getting fixated on patterns.

◉ Small bells (purchased from craft stores) can be sewn around the cover so that the elastic will ring when it is shaken. While this addition can add a dimension of fun, it can also be problematic for autistic people who have a fixation with metal.

Masks

Aim

A mask transforms its wearer and provides a way of getting out of oneself, experimenting with being someone or something else.

Description

Activities with masks are most likely to be enjoyed by co-operative participants with good eyesight. Others will find the unusual feeling of wearing a mask over their head and eyes too uncomfortable. Masks should be easy to fit over the head and not too tight around the eyes.

BreakOut members enjoyed creating their own bird masks for a dance about birds in the environment-themed festival 'The Return of the Kingfisher'.

Creative improvisations on the theme of birds

During improvisation about birds in preparation for our part in an outdoor community celebration, 'The Return of the Kingfisher Festival', many of our students participated enthusiastically and creatively in the creation of 'bird solos'. The introductory activities for this improvisation included telling of the story of the return of the Kingfisher bird and a site visit, where participants explored the bush home of 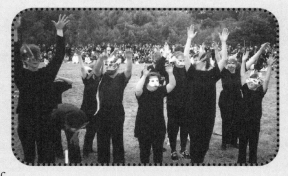 the Kingfisher. Many students developed their own choreographic ideas, transforming their body shapes into those of birds, creating bird sounds and responding to other 'birds' in a bird-like manner, pecking, scratching, waddling and flapping.

Ros, a small woman with the pear-like body shape common to adults with Down syndrome, decided that her favourite bird creature was a duck. She was lucky enough to be able to watch ducks alighting on the creek during our visit. Later, enthusiastically and authentically, Ros transformed into a waddling, pecking duck, bending forward to peck, flapping her arms that were placed on her hips as 'wings', and swivelling her hips to create a 'waddle'. Like many other people with Down syndrome, Ros had a very mobile body. Her favourite movements were full and free-flowing hip swivels, a kind of movement signature that appeared in many of her improvisations. These swivels made Ros an enchanting and convincing duck.

Make your own mask:
Equipment
Vaseline, medical plaster bandaging (available from pharmacies), elastic, scissors, bowl of water, found objects such as feathers, leaves, flowers, gumnuts, paint and brushes for decoration.

First session
◉ Prepare participant's face by rubbing Vaseline all around the eyes, eyebrows, bridge of the nose and temples to prevent plaster from sticking.

◉ Tear plaster bandages into small strips (approximately 8 cm x 3 cm long).

◉ Dip bandage strips into a bowl of water, one at a time, then while the participant holds their face really still, apply the strips to the brow, temple and eye socket area, overlaying like papier-mâché. Keep bandages away from the eyes and hairline.

◉ Just before the bandages dry, gently loosen the mask from the face and lift it off.

◉ Before it is completely dry, make a small hole in each side of the mask for elastic fastening.

Second session
Leave mask until it is fully dry – at least a couple of days later – then trim to even the edges and make comfortable for the wearer. Decorate with feathers and natural objects, such as flowers, gumnuts and leaves. Paint can be added to fill in gaps and give an overall colour. Thread elastic through the side holes and tie it to fit comfortably tightly around the head. A touch of paint to match hair colour can make the elastic less visible.

Music
To create an other-worldy atmosphere, choose music such as
◉ Jean-Michel Jarre (1993), *Oxygene*
◉ David Bowie, *2001: A Space Odyssey.*

Parachute

Parachute activities are most suitable for able adults or older children. They are also lovely for adults and children to do together, perhaps on a day when parents visit the dance class, or when there are lots of volunteers.

The most important aspect of working with a parachute is the fun of it. Its sheer size and the magical quality of the fabric make it irresistible, even to the most unengaged students. It is also a very easy means of including a whole group in a single activity.

Where can you get parachutes?
Real parachutes can be purchased from army disposal stores. However, these can be difficult for young children or older adults to manipulate and require a very large space with high ceilings. Smaller, more manageable parachutes, specially made for this kind of activity can be purchased from educational suppliers. A car cover made of silky fabric is an adequate substitute for a real parachute.

Creating waves to go under

Aims

Group togetherness, co-operation, timing, new experiences of moving.

Description

The group stands evenly spaced around the parachute, holding it in their hands. With an up-and-down movement of their hands, participants create small 'waves' with the fabric.

Singly, or in twos or small groups, participants run in under the 'waves', creating their own movement response to the fluid, floaty, windy space.

Music

Something floaty and wave-like, such as:

◎   Vivaldi, *Four Seasons*

◎   James Galway, *Songs of the Seashore*

◎   Tony O'Connor (1996), *Sea Australia*.

Creating clouds to go over

Aims

New sensory experiences, developing strong, slow movements.

Description

Group members stand spaced evenly around the parachute, holding it in their hands. Everyone squats or kneels down, making ripply wave movements with the fabric.

Participants singly, or in small groups, step in onto 'clouds', experimenting with the feeling of walking on the rippling fabric. This is a challenging movement experience because of the apparently unstable ground. The changing shape of the parachute requires strong slow movements.

Spinning in circles

Aim

For developing group co-operation.

Description

Group members stand evenly spaced around the outside of the parachute, holding the edge in their hands. Begin by walking slowly around in a circle, gradually increasing speed. Members who prefer slow movements can be encouraged to experience speed in this activity. It is important to increase speed slowly as this activity can get out of control easily.

Variation

Change speed or direction, eg slow down, speed up, forwards and backwards, clockwise and anti-clockwise.

Under the dome

Aim

This is a lovely quiet way to finish a session.

Description

Group members stand around the edges of parachute, waving it slowly up and down, making larger and larger waves. When the parachute reaches a very high point, the whole group pulls it down sharply towards the ground. As the parachute comes down everyone runs in and under the dome quickly, to sit or lie down on the inside edge of the parachute. With practice, this can produce a very slowly deflating dome that feels first like an igloo, then like a silk cover. With the whole group inside it, this can create a cosy and magical sense of togetherness.

Ribbon sticks

Short ribbon sticks

Aim

These can be useful movement activities for people who are chair-bound, or as part of a warm-up or on the spot activity.

Description

The extension of the body provided by the ribbon, as well as the visual interest in the movement of colour and pattern, helps participants go beyond their comfort zone, focus their attention on their own movement or that of others. They can also be used in relaxation or quieter body awareness activities if they are fluttered over different body parts of a participant, drawing attention to each part in turn.

How to make short ribbon sticks

Short ribbon sticks can be made by pinning a small bunch of ribbons each about 50 cm long and 1 cm wide to the head of a chopstick.

Long ribbon sticks, like those used in Chinese traditional dances, can be made by attaching satin ribbons approximately 1 m x 10 cm to a piece of dowel or bamboo. Wonderful flowing movement patterns can be created by connecting the ribbon to the stick by a fishing swivel (available from fishing supply shops).

Long ribbon sticks

Aim

Ribbon sticks, like those used in Chinese traditional dances, can be especially successful in motivating students to move through space and extend their movement, as the size and weight of the ribbons necessitates large, strong actions.

Description

There are endless possibilities for movement patterns with ribbons. A good introductory activity can begin with the group leader demonstrating and naming patterns, such as:

- figure 8
- zig-zags
- loops and circles
- streaming (participants travel fast and allow the ribbon to stream out behind them)
- question and answer (one participant responds to their partner's movement),
- canon (participants repeat same movement in sequence after each other).

Music

Something fun and lively, such as:

- *Strictly Ballroom Soundtrack,* Track: 'Love Is In The Air'
- Or with a more Chinese flavour: K.C. Wang (1996), *Chinese Bamboo Flute Songs*
- Putumayo World Music, *Tea Lands*.

Including other dance styles: folk and social dance

This section describes four folk-style dances that have been danced and enjoyed by BreakOut members. There are many other possibilities. Organisations that can provide further resources and information are listed in Appendix D.

Folk dance

Folk dance can provide an interesting contrast to creative dance, as it is quite the opposite aesthetic, in that steps and formations are set and performed in a pre-determined sequence. A version of an Irish set dance is described below. We created it in response to group members' interest in the phenomenon of 'Riverdance', a popularised form of traditional Irish dance.

Irish set-dance 'Riverdance'

Irish music lends itself well to set dances, performed in groups of around eight people (four couples arranged longways). Participants in these kinds of dances have the opportunity to enjoy working as a couple, and as part of a larger group.

Starting position: Four couples face each other in a longways set:

X   X (top couple)

X   X

X   X

X   X (bottom couple)

Patterns

- *All in, all out:* Dancers face their own partner, walk towards them, greeting each other perhaps with a nod of the head or a boisterous 'Hello!', then walk backwards to their original position
- *Do-si-do*: Partners travel towards each other, passing right shoulders, circling around each other without changing direction and then return to their original place backwards.
- *Arming:* Partners link elbows and spin together on the spot, before returning to original place or changing sides of the set with their partner.

- ⑥ *Archways*: The top couple hold hands and form an archway. All other couples walk or gallop up to the top of the set, go under that archway, then peel off (partner on the left turning to the left and partner on the right turning to the right, to walk down to the bottom of the set), perhaps go under another archway there, and then re-form.

- ⑥ *Finish:* Bow to your partner.

Music
Riverdance soundtrack.

Folk dance provides a window into other cultures

The historical and cultural functions of folk dance include reinforcing a sense of community and provision of opportunities for physical and social contact between same and opposite sex dancers. These intentions are useful for groups that include people with disabilities. Folk dance can also provide a window into different cultures, as the following story tells.

Russian dance connects with Stefan's Russian heritage

One day the adult class at BreakOut were dancing a slow and graceful Russian dance, 'Weseni Chorovod'. This is one of the oldest and most original forms of Russian dance, performed mostly by women to celebrate spring. The father of group member Stefan came a little late to drop him off that day and stayed to watch this dance with great interest. When we finished, he explained that watching the dance had brought back memories of his early years in Russia.

The footwork for this dance is very simple, comprising slow sets of walking steps. Despite its simplicity, the dance is interesting because of the patterns created as the group walks, including spirals, concentric circles and a snail. It has a surprise ending, as the final pattern takes the group into a series of twists and archways to create a kind of tunnel that magically unwinds as the dance finishes.

Dance instructions, music and a video of this dance are available from AVDP World Dance (see contact details in the Appendix D).

Folk dance offers experiences of different movement patterns

Dancing together as part of a large group offers opportunities for leadership and co-operation and experiences of new patterns and directions for moving through space. This can be both enjoyable and a challenge, especially for those people who find co-operation and physical contact difficult. One dance we have enjoyed offers all of these experiences.

Zorba's dance – dancing anti-clockwise in shoulder hold

The infamous Zorba's Dance, a popular form of the traditional Greek syrtaki, is danced in a semi-circle, with dancers connected in a shoulder hold. This positioning contrasts with the holds of the set dance of the Anglo-Celtic traditions, which requires people to physically connect only by an occasional touch of hand or elbows. Travel patterns are different too. In Greek circle dances, participants always move anti-clockwise, following the leadership of the person at the head of the line, while in set dances, travel patterns are mostly forward and backward steps.

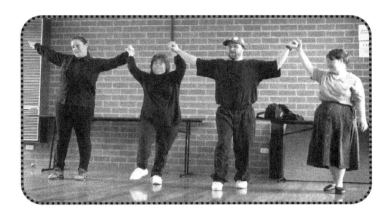

Starting position

Dancers stand in a line with arms in shoulder hold (i.e. arms laid along the neighbour's upper arms). Leader stands on far right end of the line.

- *Footwork:* Three steps travelling clockwise (R, L, R) and lift L leg; step to left on L and lift R leg; repeat throughout the music. This step speeds up and slows down with the music
- *Direction of travel:* Dance travels anti-clockwise
- *Facing direction:* Dancers face into centre of circle.

Variation
Simple version
- Step on R, L, R, pause; step on L, pause; repeat.
- Hold: Instead of shoulder hold, dancers connect by holding hands.

Complex version
- Patterns: The leader can make even simple steps interesting by leading the group all around the space, varying direction and travel pattern.
- Finish position: The leader brings group to make small circle, all facing in.

Music
- Traditional version: soundtrack, *Zorba the Greek*
- Disco version: LCD (1998), *Zorba's Dance.*

Folk dance provides an easy way to include visitors and outsiders

Folk dance is also an easy and enjoyable activity for including outsiders in a dance experience. At BreakOut, we often schedule a folk-dance at the end of our performances as a way of extending the enjoyment of dance to families and friends in attendance.

Visitors join BreakOut performers for Lambada dance

One year we had a Lambada (Latin-style line dance) as our finale. BreakOut dancers performed the whole piece first, demonstrating solos, partner and group sequences they had created in class. Then the music was repeated and the performers gradually made their way off-stage in a line formation. One class member took the role as leader, and the rest of the class followed, connecting themselves to the person in front by placing their hands on that person's waist. As the dancers passed members of the audience they knew, they left the line, invited that person to join in the dance by taking their hand and reconnecting with the line. By the end of the piece, we had most of the audience joined up in our Lambada lines.

Music

Bando Tropicana E Benedito Costa (1987), *Lambada Latin Disco.*

Popular dances

Popular dances with set steps offer another kind of enjoyable shared experience for class members. Some of these dances we have used in classes include such old favourites as 'The Hokey Pokey', 'The Chicken' or 'Little Bird Dance', 'The Mexican Hat Dance', and more recent favourites including 'The Bus-Stop', 'The Nutbush' and 'The Macarena'.

Music for these kind of dances is easily obtainable on CD disco compilations, like *The Bird Dance and Other Party Favourites* (1998).

Social dancing

Dancing as a couple using specific moves and body positioning provides another enjoyable kind of movement experience.

Strictly Ballroom: Ballroom dancing provides an opportunity for interaction with visitors

The final item of our performance of the musical *Strictly Ballroom* was a partner dance in ballroom style. The music for this dance begins with the slow and romantic 'Love is In The Air', which flows into the more lively paced 'Yesterday's Hero'. The piece began with our performers demonstrating their prowess as partners dancing together, before the MC gave the instruction to 'change partners'. At this point, each dancer had to go out into the audience and invite a visitor friend to dance. The class members' recently acquired skills in positioning themselves in ballroom hold, meant that they could guide new partners into position if necessary and lead the dance. Then as the music gradually hotted up with 'Yesterday's Hero', people were already comfortably partnered up and were able to relax into more free-form social dancing.

Enriching the dance process with other art forms

A creative dance program can be enriched through other art forms including music, drama, visual arts, film-making and creative writing. These mediums have the capacity to energise dance, as well as encourage a richer form of self-expression in participants. Activities in these artforms also offer participants opportunities to establish relationships with artists outside the disability culture.

At BreakOut we have been fortunate over the years to have group leaders, assistants, students and volunteers with other areas of expertise including visual art, music and theatre training. We have drawn on their skills in regular sessions by asking these people to lead specific activities, such as a drama game for warm-up or a drawing exercise for closure. We also regularly employ artist/s to conduct special workshops in their artforms. These have been exciting occasions when previously unrecognised talents have been discovered, imaginations have been energised and new skills developed.

The visit of an artist also creates an opportunity for a group leader to step back from their leadership role and interact with the group as a participant, as well as to observe the engagement of group members. It can also provide a chance to develop new skills and inspire new ways of facilitating dance and movement. Visiting artists bring with them expertise from their particular art form and can make complex tasks from their specialist area appear simple, fun and inspiring. Employing a skilled artist is the best way to venture into new territory for the first time.

The following section describes some of the special events we have offered at BreakOut and the value of them for members.

Music, dance and storytelling

BreakOut and Wild Moves African Drummers

A workshop with Melbourne-based African drumming and dance group Wild Moves was one such exciting event. This group has a particular style of teaching drumming through storytelling, relating the drumming rhythm to its place of origin. The BreakOut workshop was Wild Moves' first experience of working with people with intellectual disabilities, and they had expressed some concern about the appropriateness of their teaching style for engaging the group. After a preliminary discussion, it was decided that Wild Moves would proceed as they would with any group but at a slower pace and using simplified instructions.

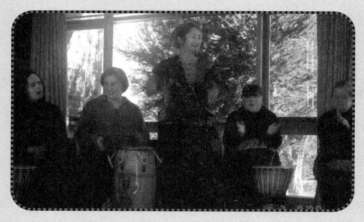

Wild Moves brought with them a collection of African drums and Ghanian fabrics. The drums were placed in a circle and each participant chose a piece of fabric to wear as a way of entering into the cultural experience. Once each BreakOut member was positioned at a drum and dressed in brightly coloured traditional material, the head drummer began by telling a story that explained how particular rhythms came to life, while another Wild Move member danced the story. This story was completely captivating to BreakOut members and for its duration there was not a distracted person in the room. This was a significant achievement for BreakOut members, given the African accent of the story teller and the length of time they had to sit still and listen. This marvellous introduction highlighted the power of theatre and storytelling to capturing the imagination of participants.

The introductory story was followed by the head drummer playing a rhythm that was repeated by BreakOut members. His first simple rhythms gradually became more complex. A number of participants excelled at replicating the difficult rhythms, to everyone's surprise. The lead drummer introduced new rhythms with clarity that enabled participants to change from one rhythm to another. His skill in doing this gave the group confidence that increased excitement levels and inspired their commitment to the task of drumming.

continued

In the second part of the workshop, some members chose to dance while others continued to drum. The live music created an intensity of focus on the dance as it had with the drumming. There was a heightened level of physical alertness, group focus and strength in movement in all the people who danced. The energy was contagious and it was a case of having to stop so that people could go home rather than wanting to stop. Even the hall cleaner put down her broom, joined the group and was swept away by the excitement of the music!

This workshop inspired one BreakOut member to buy her own drum and other members were eager to play the group leader's drum regularly in class. For many months afterwards, drumming was a favoured activity of all participants. By the end of the year, the members of BreakOut's older adult group were so at ease with playing drums that we constructed a performance piece based on the drumming circle. This activity brought focus, energy and dignity to an otherwise low-energy and often disconnected group. One of the most memorable and surprising outcomes of this workshop was the discovery that the introductory story told by the drumming leader was remembered and referred to many times afterwards by the participants. It was an experience that reminded us not to underestimate the cognitive and imaginative capacity of people with intellectual disabilities.

Drama and dance

Creating a musical play *Strictly Ballroom*

I (Kim) was working with a class of teenagers with mild intellectual disabilities in an expressive drama/dance program. We had decided to create a performance as a focus for the semester's work, to be attended by families and fellow students from the school. We bandied about several ideas for this event, experimenting with improvised movement and dialogue, but found ourselves lacking continuity and a strong sense of purpose.

One day someone came to class excited about having seen the current movie hit, *Strictly Ballroom.* This discussion immediately sparked some ideas from class members and myself, most of whom had recently seen the movie. A ballroom dance theme seemed a perfect choice for a class that comprised roughly even numbers of boys and girls, and the script would provide a stepping off place for both drama and dance work. We began to devise a simple script based on the story and to interweave dialogue with choreography.

Together, the class and I (Kim) watched the movie, discussing our favourite parts and characters and the reasons we liked them. The words that students used to describe their reasons for liking particular characters or moments included 'great costumes,

continued

funny jokes, romantic, loud, silly'. We talked about which roles students would prefer to take on and how they could see themselves or each other as particular characters. Then we began the process of creating our own *Strictly Ballroom,* by whittling down the script to a few key scenes and auditioning for the characters in those scenes.

Those students who wanted a speaking part needed to have the capacity to remember dialogue and be able to reproduce it loudly enough for an audience to hear. Those who wanted romantic parts needed to be able to remember sequences well enough to enable co-operative performance with a partner. Everyone who took a major role needed to be committed to the ongoing process of rehearsal and then public performance. Some group decisions had to be made and people had to abide by those, even when the decision was not made in their favour.

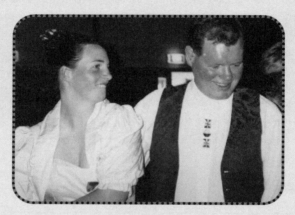

Group member Steve, who took the part of MC Barry Fyffe, delivered his welcoming remarks competently in the presence of our class, but as soon as another person came into the theatre it became more difficult for him. Fortunately our audience on the big day was very supportive and allowed Steve several false starts before he managed the lines well enough to get the show underway. This introduction was met with thunderous applause. I am hopeful that the memory of that positive response may overlay Steve's fears about being in front of an audience and perhaps help him with his next big performance.

The pairings for the ballroom dances had been worked out as best we could, with those who needed more support paired up with those who were able to remember and perform under pressure. On the day of the show, Kylie was particularly out of sorts when she was forced to abide by a group decision about costuming that didn't suit her. Her ill-humour worsened as the event progressed, and by the time the final big number came along, Kylie would not take hands with the eager young man who was expecting her and instead paired up with her favourite class member. This meant that the two performers who did not meet the partner they had expected were left forlornly wandering the floor at the climactic moment. The strongest verbal cues from stage right about 'pairing up' were not picked up. Eventually the pattern was put to rights with some swift co-active positioning by a teacher's assistant, who took the lost sheep by the hand and got them together.

continued

There were many challenges for students in this undertaking, with dialogue, action and dance sequences to learn. No class members had the capacity to cope with all of these at the same time as learning some strategies for coping with the unexpected. So when things went wrong, they really went wrong!

The most charming scene was the romantic rhumba, 'Dance of Love'. Paul and Jane were good friends to begin with and were well matched as the romantic lover–dancers, Fran and Scott. They were both thrilled to have won those roles and were equally committed to their duet that required memory work, some on-the-spot improvisation and considerable co-operation. At times when Paul was a little shaky, he was helped by forthright verbal and physical cues from the more confident Jane. This performance was a very memorable moment for both young people and their families who attended.

Ian McCurrach and Barbara Darnley's book *Special Needs: Special Talents* (1999) offers a wealth of information on this topic.

Film-making

BreakOut makes a film

Introduction: The project

BreakOut assisted me (Jenny) to produce a dance piece for a choreographic project which was a requirement of my graduate dance and movement training (GMD). This was to be shown for assessment to university staff, as well as students and invited guests. The project required BreakOut to step into a non-disability culture and interact with the wider community on many levels.

The idea was to make a black and white film that would capture the human face of the BreakOut dancers, to be projected onto the performance space behind the dancers as they were performing. I approached Natalie Poole, a fellow dance student who was also a film-maker, with the idea of a collaborative project. Natalie was interested in the project because she had not previously worked with people with an intellectual disability and, as a dancer, was curious about their dance skills.

The project was to have three elements: film, dance and performance. It was important that the film be visually engaging for an audience and complement the movement of the dancers. We also had a very small budget and basic equipment that ruled out editing or any complex technical production. We decided to work with Super 8 film so we would need only a basic projector, and not expensive video technology. Super 8 projection also has the advantage that it can be manually manipulated to speed up or slow down.

continued

Film concept

Once the decisions were made about how we would make the film, we then needed to decide what to film. We had recently had a conversation at BreakOut, prompted by comments from one of the more independent and vocal members of the group, about her feelings of frustration at not being able to do things she sees other people doing, such as getting married, driving a car and having different jobs. As a group, we took this feeling into an image and explored it further. Firstly we imagined ourselves locked inside a box - what we would do to get out and how it would feel once we were out. This seemed to be a promising possibility to be explored for a film and dance piece. This concept provided lots of scope for developing movements with contrasting dynamics such as strength to express anger and frustration and flow to express freedom. The imaginary boxes became real boxes, ones big enough for us to climb in and out of. We decided to call the piece 'Boxes'.

Natalie attended a session while we were still in the improvisation phase of the dance. This gave her the opportunity to see people when they were less self-conscious about performance and to capture more spontaneous expression. Her impending visit on Week 4 of an eight-week project brought new energy and enthusiasm to members.

The film-making process

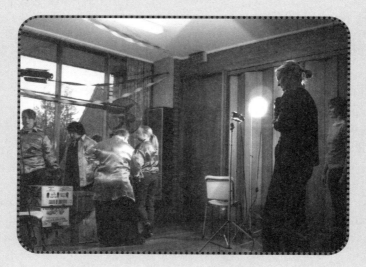

Making the film was a new experience for all of us. The special lighting required for the film meant that we had to contain all our movements within a section of the space. This was challenging, as group members were used to moving without restriction in regular BreakOut sessions. The presence of new people and equipment contributed to a general feeling of excitement, as well as difficulty in keeping people focused. After recognising the challenges group members were facing, we decided to sit down and

continued

have a discussion about the basics of film-making, such as the camera's need for light. Natalie then demonstrated how the room changed with the lights on. She then showed us her camera and gave each person an opportunity to look through the lens. We then looked at the area on the ground that was lit up by the lights and asked members to walk around the edge of the lit-up area to define the dance space more clearly. After these explanations, the group became more focused on the task and their excitement was directed into dancing. Over the course of the hour and half session, Natalie captured 3.5 minutes of appealing moments that became 'the film'.

The performance

For the performance, the film was projected on a screen at the side of the performance space. The dancers stood behind their boxes in the darkened room. The film was played as the opening to the piece, while the stage area remained in darkness. Once the film was finished, the lights came up and the dance began.

Re-working the performance

After the show, we thought back over this process and decided that this had perhaps not been the best way of integrating the two mediums. Later in the year, we had the opportunity to re-work the piece for another performance that was to take place on a traditional stage with a white backdrop. This meant that the film could be projected onto the backdrop behind the dancers. Instead of having the film play only as an introduction, we decided to slow down the projection speed so that the film played in slow motion throughout the piece. This meant that the film images and the real life people were dancing together and had the effect of bringing the audience even closer to experiencing the people, their personalities and their dance.

Outcomes

Creating a film gave BreakOut members the opportunity to work with a skilled film-maker and explore a medium new to all of us. We learnt that new experiences like this needed time for introduction and explanation, and that change to the program's usual routine needed to be accommodated. Group members learnt some basic concepts about film-making experientially, and enjoyed the opportunity to be 'film stars'. Natalie was excited about the range of human expression she was able to capture through the eye of the camera. This had a positive effect on the way she engaged with the group and inspired her to explore further opportunities to work with people with intellectual disabilities. One of the benefits of having made a film is that, unlike dance, which is so ephemeral, film can provide a valuable source of documentation that lasts indefinitely.

Creative Writing

BreakOut and the poet's pen

My (Jenny's) idea of using a poem to accompany a performance piece led to a request to a poet friend, Christopher Brown, to create a poem based on thoughts and feelings of group members. I felt comfortable asking Christopher to assist because of his writing skills, and because he had attended BreakOut classes a number of times and had enjoyed dancing with the group. I felt confident that he would be inspired by the group's ideas and would also enjoy the challenge of using the group's own words to create a poem to tell their story.

The group's discussion on the performance theme of 'Landscapes' generated many ideas from members, including:
◉ special places, such as the beach, the desert, the park
◉ special people in their lives, such as boyfriends, parents and grandparents
◉ animals and favourite colours.

When asked how these special places made them feel, one person sang 'Do Re Me' from the *Sound of Music* in a very animated voice. This response made it obvious that her special place made her feel happy. Another person spoke about feeling free.

As the group workshopped ideas for the performance, so many personal experiences and feelings were generated that we felt both the written and spoken word would complement the dance. With permission from the group, I then sent these ideas to Christopher for him to use as the raw material for the poem. When it was completed, the next session began with a reading of the poem. Group members quickly identified with the parts of the poem that had originally been theirs by smiling, laughing or saying 'that's me'. The poem worked to affirm people's feelings.

At the end-of-year performance the poem was read out by Tabetha, a group member assisted by me. It was a touching moment for the audience as they witnessed this young woman with an intellectual disability stand with pride in front of the audience and give voice to the thoughts and feelings of her peers. Some audience members commented that it was helpful to them to have articulated in words the ideas behind the dance.

Landscapes of Colour

If I could fly in wings and ride,
The coloured landscapes deep inside.
To touch the treasures of my heart,
Its joys, its sorrows, memories art.
To hold and be held in that place
Ones I love and see their face.
Father, an aunt, sunbeams turn yellow;

continued

Mother's red lips, sweet kiss, so mellow.
A place that's tinged with deeper blue,
Grandfather's passing, sadder hue.
Flushing pink when my boyfriend holds my hand,
Dancing at parties and feeling so grand.
The "Sound of Music", bright colours bring,
"Doe, Ray, Me" raises a joyous ring.
Green places of freedom, my special space,
Being with myself, finding my own pace.
To draw in bright orange the people I love,
And dance with warm colours held high above.
Always knowing I can come and be,
With friends at "BreakOut" and feel so free.

If I could fly on wings of love,
And see a landscape from above.
To reach its colours through each cloud,
And paint their pictures clear and loud.
With yellow brush so clear and bright,
Painting sun, moon, sand, and ducks in flight.
And with a lovely light green hue,
To paint the grass so fresh and new.
And then with colour darker green,
I sketch fairies their wings with sheen.
My flight continues northward spread,
Capturing Uluru's Rock in vivid red.

Through clouds I drift with orange brush,
I gently wash the sunset's blush.
When orange dabs with red, it's loud,
More like a carrot than a cloud.
Flight's end finds now St Kilda beach,
With blue I work the watery reach.
And its sands my rest I make,
My coloured wings the seagulls take.

Landscapes of colour, pure delight,
Join our voyage, enjoy your flight.

Poem reprinted with the kind permission of Christopher Brown

Chapter 6

Creating a performance

Introducing performance

Performing in front of an audience can be an enjoyable and inspiring experience. Performing combinations can be as varied as solos, duets, small and large groups, performing in front of possible audiences of one other person, a class of peers, a supportive group of friends and family or a large audience of strangers. All of these opportunities offer different experiences for the performer that are mostly, but not always, positive. Sometimes the added intensity of the presence of an audience can inspire extra achievements or a moment of magic. At other times, performers who are ill-prepared or not skilled enough can be disadvantaged by a public performance.

For people with intellectual disabilities, the possible benefits of performing are likely to be roughly equivalent with the level of support needs. Thus, while many people with mild intellectual disabilities will be stimulated by the experience of performing, a focus on performance outcomes in a dance program for clients with high support needs is unlikely to be appropriate.

In this chapter we discuss the possible benefits of performing, a variety of performing options and several models for creating dance performances.

Outcomes of performing

The process of performing can have positive outcomes for individual participants that include development of leadership skills and creative transformation. It can also have the more political outcome of enhancing family and community perceptions of people with disabilities.

The following section also discusses issues about performing in public, the risks and the benefits.

Development of leadership skills

Performing offers opportunities for participants to develop leadership skills. This can be as simple as leading an activity in class, for example, one movement in the warm up (such as 'Make your own move', as described in Chapter 2), or it can be as challenging as taking responsibility for a section or item in a public performance.

An entry in the journal that I (Jenny) kept during my graduate dance studies describes my pleasure in the development of leadership skills of BreakOut's young adult group.

I enjoy seeing the heightened level of focus and engagement between members that has developed over time. It is possible with this level of engagement to hand over leadership to group members, thus offering them opportunities to lead the group in their own style. This is my ideal. When this is achieved within a group, we become a team and my facilitation is there primarily to support the group.

The following story describes the significance to BreakOut member Jon of a performing experience in which he and classmate Julia enjoyed a leadership experience through dance.

Julia and Jon fly with Renee and Ellie

One day I (Jenny) brought a bag of scarves that I had not used for some time to class. As each participant chose their favourite, Jon picked up a sparkly black and gold scarf and commented, 'This reminds me of BreakOut Concert 1998' (some four years and many performances earlier). At first, I could not remember the event to which Jon referred. He reminded me of the piece in which he and classmate Julia had given a 'floating cloud ride' to tiny children Ellie and Renee, at the beginning of their dance 'Stars'. I thought back to this performance and remembered how Jon and Julia had seemed to really enjoy the responsibility, remembering and managing their props well, being very careful of the children and how they had been very proud of the positive audience response. The children in turn had given themselves over with great trust and comfort to the magic ride. It seemed that this event had made a big impact on Jon, given how well he recalled it four years later.

Creative transformation through performance

Involvement in creative arts performance offers experiences that are beyond the scope of other recreational activities. The sense of transformation afforded by being outside one's everyday self is usually very pleasurable. Those who have felt the high that usually follows an on-stage experience will know that it can be very intense. The power of transformation achieved through performance, especially when shared with friends, families and peers has been well documented. People in a range of circumstances, for example, with people with intellectual (Schlusser, 2000) and physical disabilities (Benjamin, 2001), female prisoners (Dunphy, 1999), Maori cultural performers (Dunphy, 1996) and primary school students (Bond, 1994) describe the experience of transformation as a major motivating factor for participation in performing arts experiences.

The magical transformative times are the ones that make all the hard work seem worth it. One of these is described below.

Rosie waves 'goodbye'

This photo shows Rosie in one of the special moments that can occur during performances. Rosie often attends BreakOut classes without becoming more than minimally engaged in the dance, as she has autism and mostly prefers to stay in her own world. On the occasion of this performance, Rosie suddenly began to participate spiritedly in the choreography, which was about travelling and saying goodbye. The meaning of choreographing, rehearsing and performing seemed suddenly to have come to her. Rosie's face shone with delight as she said 'goodbye' with a lively wave that was returned by an enthusiastic member of the audience. The challenge on this occasion turned out not to be getting Rosie inspired, but to get her to stop dancing and leave the stage once the item ended.

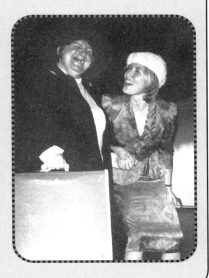

The power of performance on the audience

Ideally, it is not only the performers but the audience who experience the power of performance. A successful performance is one in which the audience has enjoyed themselves, learned something new or been especially moved. Maoris call this 'ihi' (power) and 'wehi' (spirit), the magical elements of a performance that give the audience a shiver down the spine.

Enhancing family and community perceptions of people with disabilities

As well as the personal impact on individual audience members, performances by people with intellectual disabilities can have more political outcomes through the enhancement of the role of disabled people in society. In the case of BreakOut, we have a deliberate intention to make a political statement. One of the group's aims is to 'improve community perceptions of the artistic and expressive capabilities of people with disabilities'.

A successful performance can enhance the perceptions of families, carers and disability professionals, as well as outsiders such as community centre users, festival participants and the general public. Many of these people may not otherwise have had an opportunity to think of people with intellectual disabilities as performers, or as being capable of creative artistry.

Families of children with intellectual disabilities, many of whom suffer chronic grief about the child who might have been, need opportunities to celebrate their child's achievements, perhaps even more than other parents. The following case study illustrates the positive experience of the foster mother of one young man with moderate intellectual disabilities after his performing debut.

Jason takes a leadership role through dance

I (Kim) undertook a dance artist residence at a special developmental school around the time of the lead-up to the 1996 Olympic Games. The Olympics was therefore an obvious choice for a theme for the school's performance at the Combined Special Schools Music Concert. Students created structured improvisations for individual pieces based on their favourite sports. A giant parade, like an Olympics closing ceremony, was developed as an appropriate and accessible way of including all students, even those confined to wheelchairs.

Parents who attended seemed to really enjoy the spectacle. One of those students was Jason, a large young man with Down syndrome, who exuberantly led his 'team' with a giant flag and waved boisterously to the audience from the front of the stage. Jason's foster mother cried with pride when she saw his delight in performing on stage. This was the first time she had seen him take a leadership role, and she was thrilled to see Jason managing it so competently and with so much enjoyment.

People who share community facilities with intellectually disabled performers might develop a greater awareness of the potential for people with intellectual disabilities, for example, by being in the same building at the same time and witnessing performances. At the other extreme, it is possible for the experience of seeing a performance by people with disabilities to be life-changing, as it was for me (Kim) when I saw the stunning performance of 'Stepping Out' by children with intellectual disabilities at the Sydney Opera House in 1982. This aspect of dance and theatre, hitherto unknown to me, inspired me to move towards a new life direction – firstly to dance therapy and then to community dance with people with disabilities.

Community members' perceptions of people with intellectual disabilities can be challenged quite unexpectedly, as the following story tells.

Changing a council bus depot supervisor's view of people with disabilities as performers

I (Jenny) hired a community bus from our local council to transport BreakOut members to a festival where they were to perform. The depot supervisor, expecting dancers, was quite taken aback to meet BreakOut members, men and women with intellectual disabilities, of all shapes, sizes and ages. The group obviously didn't match his expectations of dance performers at all. We figured that the process of hiring the bus and taking members to the festival may have been worth it, if nothing else than for a new understanding for this man about who could be a dancer!

The risks of performing in public: Community involvement versus perpetuation of negative stereotypes

In addition to the benefits of performing in public there are also risks. The experience of performing in public is not always positive. There are people in the community with little experience of disability, who may not share the politically correct view that all people are entitled to an equal place in the community. At one community event, a very vociferous man chose to sit near our group and make loud comments about why 'these people' should not be there and why he preferred not to see them. At that ugly moment we did seriously question our commitment to the idea of community integration and wondered whether we really had done the right thing, creating such public exposure for BreakOut members.

When other opportunities to perform present themselves, we always face the dilemma of deciding whether or not our group's involvement will be beneficial. Will the opportunity advantage our members and enhance the dignity and public standing of people with disabilities? In making a decision we are aware that, like all minorities, each person with a disability bears the burden of representing all others in the eyes of the community.

Generally, one of the great pleasures of being involved in the performing arts is the opportunity to perform and share one's achievement with others. However, it is always important to present artwork in an appropriate context. For people with intellectual disabilities this is particularly important. Occasionally we have been asked to perform at a mainstream event like a street festival. We are generally selective with this kind of invitation, as we have had less than positive experiences with uninterested audiences and the stresses of outdoor performing. Joy's (2000) booklet discusses this issue at length with regard to JustUs, a drama group for people with intellectual disabilities. JustUs staff came to the realisation that their group needed to have a repertoire of different performance items, some that were failsafe items suitable for challenging, changeable outdoor events and some more complex ones suitable for a more controlled theatre environment.

We make the decision not to participate in a community festival

Some time ago, BreakOut was invited to perform at a local community day that was to be held outdoors in a park. The event co-ordinator was very keen to have the group participate, as he felt that it would provide good publicity for us. However, we had some concerns about the likely outcome of the performance, especially as our dancers would have been in an unfamiliar environment, on a high, unstable stage (the back of a truck) with no opportunity for onsite rehearsal, at the mercy of the weather and watched by an audience of strangers who may not necessarily have been prepared for or supportive of the endeavours of performers with disabilities. After much consideration we decided not to take the risk. We could not be confident that the performance would be a successful experience for the dancers, or that it would enhance the public persona of people with disabilities.

While we have come to the point where we no longer accept performance opportunities that we think will be risky, we wonder if we are guilty of setting up barriers for people with intellectual disabilities of participating fully in community life, of not creating the 'least restrictive environment'. This is an ongoing dilemma, and one that can perhaps only be resolved when those with disabilities are a fully accepted part of the wonderful variety of people who make up our world.

The philosophical challenge posed by the opportunity to perform in mainstream events such as our local council festival faces us all the time. While philosophically we believe that people with intellectual disabilities should have the opportunity to be part of mainstream community activities, we also have to bear in mind their special needs and the importance of creating opportunities for success. Setting up a performance for intellectually disabled performers that results in them looking incompetent in front of an audience does little to enhance community perception of people's abilities. It may even serve to reinforce some people's negative prejudices. Group leaders needs to exercise judgment about the likely benefits of opportunities that present themselves before making the decision to participate.

Performance possibilities

At BreakOut, we provide a range of graduated opportunities for performance, beginning with the least challenging. These include:

- in-class improvisation or prepared pieces shared with other group members
- occasional 'work-in-progress' showings for visitors
- an annual performance attended by audiences of supportive family and friends, clients and staff from the disability sector
- participation in larger community events for our more independent and skilled performers.

In-class performance

To introduce people with intellectual disabilities to the concept of performing it is advisable to begin with a low-risk strategy. This could be as simple as offering class members the chance to lead one movement of warm-up or one activity in class, or to perform in front of their class peers as a solo performer or as part of a duo or small group.

Schlusser documents the practice of in-class performance that she has refined with her Stretch Theatre Company of adults with intellectual disabilities. She comments on performers' enjoyment of the process as evidenced by their 'readiness to perform, passionate involvement in the process of performing and pleasure in the applause' (2000, p. 111). In-class performance is an intermediary step that is valuable for introducing the frightening, exhilarating feeling of 'butterflies in the stomach' that comes with facing an audience.

The following story about group member Veronica describes her progress as a performer over 18-months of weekly dance sessions.

Veronica finds her way to centre stage

Veronica is a member of a creative dance program I (Jenny) lead at an adult training service. Veronica lives much of her life through her imagination, referring to herself as a princess or a mermaid and describing imaginary adventurous things she has done like crocodile hunting and swimming with Flipper the dolphin. Her imagination is so active it is difficult for her to maintain focus on any group activity.

Veronica's dance group's weekly three-hour session includes time for a short solo performance from each participant. Veronica has loved the idea of this opportunity, but found it difficult to carry out successfully. In the beginning, she would make her choice of music enthusiastically, position herself in a corner of the room and then just smile to herself as she dreamed away to the music. After some weeks, she began to move her arms in wide circles and say, 'Wow' a few times during her piece of music. Months later Veronica began to develop some movement expression, but still remained mostly in her own world with little sense of sharing or performing for the group.

After some time, I decided that it was important for Veronica to become more spatially aware as a way of developing some connection with the audience and to prompt a move from her contained world in the corner. I marked out squares on the floor with masking tape and strategically placed them so that she came closer to the audience with every step into a new square. Veronica was delightfully surprised to find herself close to the audience when she stepped into the last square.

The turning point for Veronica came when she noticed her peers watching as she made her special circling arm movements and said her usual, 'Wow'. From that session on, she began to extend her sense of performance. It was as if she had needed to become aware of her potential for creating pleasure in others for this transformation to take place. Once the 'light' was switched on, Veronica began use the whole length of her selected piece of music to explore movement. Over time, her attention to the performance task improved, along with a noticeable development in her ability to dance for longer periods before disconnecting, and attending to unrelated things or wandering back to her corner.

In a recent session, Veronica started her dance in a chosen pose, used the entire performance space, created dramatic moments with balancing poses, performed fast and slow twirling movements and ended by throwing her arms up in the air saying 'Wow'. She followed this dance with a bow to her enthusiastic audience and remained in the performance space smiling at her peers. Veronica's development as a performer over this time confirmed for me the value of opportunities for performance, even for group members like Veronica, who initially show a lack of ability or interest. It seemed worth waiting 18 months for that moment!

Public performances

Working together to create a more formal performance can be very enjoyable, providing group members with a shared sense of purpose and focus. Open Days at BreakOut are held occasionally, at the usual time in the usual venue, functioning as a way of showing the group's in-class activities to families and carers and for those interested to follow the progress of individuals. A typical Open Day session might include warm-up and improvisation sections, as well as work in progress, i.e. performance items that are being developed.

BreakOut's annual performance is a more formal affair, held in a professional setting in community theatre. Sometimes the stage is used, but at other times all action takes place on the theatre floor, allowing for a larger performing area and less difficulty with performers having to manage steps, stage wings, the darkness and unfamiliar spaces. This is an attractive option when we have members in wheelchairs, given the inaccessibility of the stage.

Mostly audiences at BreakOut events are familiar with people who have intellectual disabilities, and are very supportive, whatever the outcome. Sometimes items prepared very carefully work out as planned but there are other times when they don't. The stories below exemplify the two extremes. The first is an example of a carefully rehearsed event that was not successful, while the second details a completely unexpected and very gratifying breakthrough that occurred during a performance.

Act It Out performance goes off!

The first time I (Kim) worked with one group of teenagers from a special school we created an original play, 'Steve Bryce goes to London', based on students' ideas about adventures of an Australian backpacker overseas. These students had been reasonably co-operative and focused during the rehearsal period, but on the day of the show, were disappointingly out of control. They forgot their lines, lost their characters, used their own names, and laughed and bantered with each other throughout the performance. Fortunately the audience was a supportive group of parents who were aware of the challenges for me and their young people in successfully presenting a play, so they were complimentary despite what I considered to be an unsatisfactory outcome.

The next time I created a show with this group, we began the performance with a candle dance to focus their attention (described in more detail in Chapter 5), and the show had a much more successful outcome. We were able to retrieve our pride and regenerate an understanding of the contribution of dance and drama to the education of these young people.

Carlos 'breaks out' during a BreakOut performance

The following excerpt from my (Jenny's) journal notes shows my observations of Carlos, a 30-year-old man with a moderate intellectual disability and no verbal language, over his first year of involvement in the BreakOut program. It also describes a transformation that occurred during Carlos's first public performance.

Carlos does not speak but occasionally lets out a yell, especially if he is feeling excited or agitated. He has limited access to the movement quality of flow in his body and in space, and little flexibility in his torso and lower body. Carlos' arms and face are also held in a state of rigidity. It takes a lot of 'one-to-one' engagement with him to bring him into the circle. When he does enter, he responds with random movements that mostly have a jerky quality. With assistance, Carlos will move through space, but all his movements are bound and direction is linear.

At the BreakOut performance, Carlos 'broke out' through dance and was somehow able to release movements I had not witnessed previously. Carlos appeared very aware of the audience, especially the area in which some special friends were sitting. His focus was directed to those friends most of the time he was on stage.

I held Carlos' hand as he stood on stage and was aware of the tension in his body, though I had the feeling he was more excited than nervous. He stood still for a while and then something happened. His legs loosened and he began to jump. At first they were small jumps with no regular rhythm but then the energy grew until he was jumping up and down to the beat of the music. When the music stopped, Carlos threw his arms and head into the air. He looked like a rock'n'roll star finishing a concert!

It was a great privilege to dance with Carlos on that day. I was able to experience the energy and life that lives in him, yet mostly remains contained in his silent, remote world. For weeks I have asked myself what was it that brought about this change. Something happened for Carlos in the excitement of the performance and the connection with friends while he was on stage. It was wonderful to witness him discovering freedom of self-expression through dance.

Participating in larger community events

Sometimes a dance group has the opportunity to perform in a more mainstream or community event. This can have numerous benefits, including the chance to showcase the ability of performers to a wider audience and the opportunity to see other groups performing. Two such events are described below.

The Art of Difference Festival

BreakOut was invited to perform at the Art of Difference, Melbourne's first performing arts festival for people with disabilities held in 2001. This event provided artists with disabilities the opportunity to perform in a professional theatre environment. For some BreakOut members, this was the most formal theatre experience they had had.

In a regular group session before the event we prepared members as much as we could by explaining that the audience would be a lot bigger than at regular BreakOut shows. Most group members had attended professional theatre performances and had some idea of the differences this performance would provide: big audience, colourful lights and a special stage. The idea of stepping into the world of the theatre created some anxiety among members, but mostly there was great excitement.

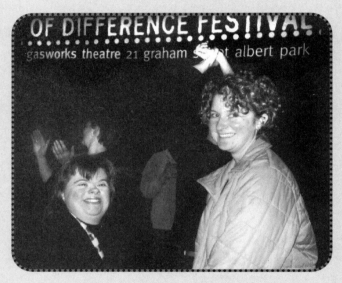

The experience was a huge success. The environment was fun, supportive and accepting. The audience was comprised of people with disabilities, carers, arts workers, professional performing artists, community groups like BreakOut, local government representatives, families and friends. The audience embraced each performance with respect and enthusiastic appreciation.

It was very dignifying to have our work and the work of other artists with disabilities valued enough to be presented in such a professional environment. The Art of Difference was an event that recognised the importance of catering for the needs of people with disabilities in order to celebrate their achievements and creativity. The organisers did not underestimate the level of physical and emotional support performers would need to assure successful participation. The festival also provided the opportunity for other community arts workers to network with each other and be affirmed in the challenging and exciting work of disability arts.

The Return of the Kingfisher Festival

We have performed several times in 'The Return of the Kingfisher Festival', a large-scale outdoor performance that celebrates the success of local environmental action. This event involves people from a large number of community and cultural groups, schools, indigenous performers and professionals and art forms as diverse as drumming, puppetry, dance and fire sculpture. Performers create their own items on a given theme. Bird improvisations, described in Chapter 1, was one such piece of choreography created by BreakOut members for the event.

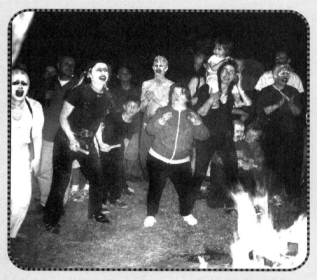

One of the most rewarding aspects of being part of such a large and inclusive event is the sense of community and achievement that is shared with other performers. As well, it is wonderful to experience from the inside, a range of different art forms. BreakOut members particularly enjoyed the drumming and chanting circle around a huge bonfire that was part of the Grand Finale of the festival. Some of the group's more confident members joined the drumming and chanting with great abandon.

When we talked about this event later, some of the factors that seemed to contribute to a highly exhilarating experience were the masks we wore, the dark, the power and warmth of the fire, the volume and hypnotic beat of drums and the physical proximity of so many involved performers.

The same aspects of this event that were so exciting also presented the greatest difficulties. It was very challenging to manage our group in such an uncontrolled environment. One member collapsed with exhaustion and had to spend the evening in a St Johns Ambulance. Another participant had a panic attack when approached by a dog, and had to be given a lot of extra attention to get through the night. After that experience we decided to invite only a selected group of the fittest and most independent members to future outdoor events.

The following section examines possible models for development of performances – some ways of generating themes and content and how these might work.

Models for creating performances

Leader-directed performances

A leader-directed performance is one that is instigated and directed by the group leader, usually to a set formula or script. This is the simplest method of creating a performance, involving selection of a theme or script that already exists and developing a show from that. Popular choices for this type of performance are musicals such as *Grease, Cats* or *The Wizard of Oz*. Choreography for shows like this are usually based on a recognised dance style, for example, rock'n'roll dance for *Grease* and ballroom dance for *Strictly Ballroom*. This makes composition easy as the set repertoire of movements and style provides the group leader with a framework for their own choreography.

Beginning with a popular story or theme means that the audience is likely to enjoy the show, even if the delivery is not faultless. It is a very suitable choice for inexperienced group leaders and performers, and/or difficult groups. And it is likely to work! The disadvantages of such an approach are that participants are not as deeply involved in the creative process and may not be stimulated to make and develop their own ideas.

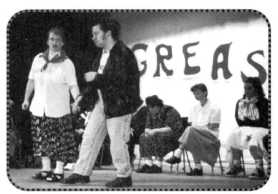

Collaborative performances

A different approach to performance is a collaborative process in which the leader guides the group through the development of their own original material. This method is suitable for leaders and groups who are ready to take on a bigger challenge, while still allowing the ultimate responsibility for success and completion of the piece to lie with the leader.

Basic steps in developing a collaborative performance

◎ Group leader and group members begin with a shared commitment to the development and production of the performance.

◎ The creative process starts with a brainstorm of ideas and themes of interest to group members.

◎ The most popular or promising theme is selected.

◎ The group generates movement ideas around this theme via a process of improvisation.

◎ Group members make choices about music, props and costumes.

◎ The group leader facilitates the creative process by leading the group through the exploration stages.

⊚ The group leader uses his/her artistic judgment to make decisions about final structure based on observations of the ideas and movements generated by members.

⊚ Members commit to group leader's decision and rehearse towards a polished end product.

The following story describes a collaborative process that BreakOut members undertook in the creation of a performance piece entitled 'Landscapes'.

'Landscapes' choreographic project

After a trip to Uluru and Central Australia, I (Jenny) returned to BreakOut excited to share all the wonderful things I had seen. During our extended 'catch-up' time, a ritual we enjoy at BreakOut after holidays, I told the group about the colours of the desert and the beauty of the red earth, blue sky and the brightly coloured flowers I had seen. I then invited members to share their thoughts about any places that were special to them.

Sometimes discussions at BreakOut can take a while to get going, but on this occasion members seemed to find no difficulty connecting with an idea or feeling about a special place, evoked by my descriptions of the desert. One person described the blue sea and seagulls at St Kilda Beach. Another member told us about her home, friends and her favourite meals. Some people named their favourite colour. Simon, a man with autism who can speak but seldom does, said very enthusiastically that his favourite colour was orange 'like the sun'.

The descriptions that emerged from this 'catch-up' time were so rich in personal meaning, that I felt compelled to use them as a starting point for our end-of-year performance. We decided to use all the colours we had spoken about to represent special places. My assistant, Vicki, and I worked out a simple structure in which colours and places were brought together to depict something of the stories people had shared. We then divided all the ideas into three sections:

Part 1: The Desert/Outback

Part 2: The Sea

Part 3: Sunshine

We decided to use fabric to represent the colours of the desert, sea and sun. I bought several four-metre-long pieces of satin, which matched the colours of the desert as closely as possible, and one-metre square pieces of satin in different shades of blue and green for the sea.

We began by creating the desert through movement. We covered the floor with the long pieces of 'desert' fabric, then walked around them to familiarise ourselves with the

continued

colours and the shapes. Then group members chose a partner and a piece of fabric to work with together, and positioned themselves at either end of the fabric, facing each other. We then had some time for improvisation. I directed this process by asking members to find ways of moving the fabric, then ways of moving their bodies with the fabric and then ways of moving the fabric and their bodies while also travelling through space. It was exciting to see how members engaged with the fabric and to witness the movement ideas that emerged. People wrapped themselves up in the fabric, one by one and simultaneously. Some people made waves so that the fabric was moved up and down and from side to side. We also played around with the element of time by moving quickly and slowly to the music. Over the following weeks, the movements created in this initial improvisation process were explored at greater depth and then worked into a structure.

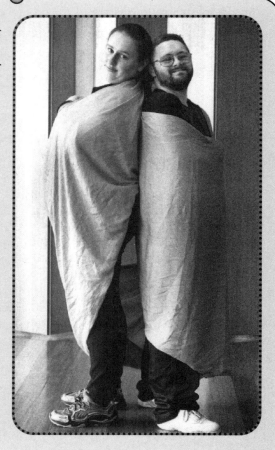

The process of bringing ideas and movements generated by the group into a structure was not difficult. It simply required listening to and observing what the group was sharing, either verbally or through movement, then highlighting those significant moments in rehearsal. For example, when two members started wrapping themselves up in the fabric so that they looked like beautiful cocoons we began to explore this movement as a group. By the end of the rehearsal process all group members were able to accomplish this task and seemed to thoroughly enjoy the feeling of the satin on their bodies and the intimacy created between themselves and their partners. This type of exploration was carried out with a number of different movements. I then decided on what would be the most visually interesting way of connecting the movements.

We had finished the 'desert' section of the performance within four weeks, so we followed a similar process to develop our dance expression for the sea and the sunshine during the last four weeks of term. We used the square pieces of blue and green fabric to represent the sea. We explored the possibility of bringing all the squares together to form one big sea, and discovered that by working as partners, it was possible to make a connecting point of fabric with another pair. Visually this looked very effective, as all

continued

the fabrics came together to form what one member described as a 'patchwork quilt sea'. This section was created simply by changing the spatial relationship between the dancers using closeness/connectedness and distance/separation as the two variables. As accompaniment we chose a piece of music that reminded us of the sounds of the sea, Tony O'Connor's *Sea Australia*.

The final part of the performance was inspired by a group member's passionate enjoyment of the song 'Walking on Sunshine'. In the rehearsal process each person contributed a movement to express the way the sun made them feel. We then put all those movements together to form a sequence that we danced to the chorus of the song. Each time we performed the dance there was a heightened level of excitement during the chorus as each person anticipated their personal movement gesture. A strong feeling of celebration emerged with this dance, so we decided to make this the final item in the performance.

After eight weeks of weekly rehearsals the piece was ready to perform. We decided to call it 'Landscapes' to capture the many places and feelings that had inspired our dance making process.

Participant-developed performances

Another method of creating a performance is the development of choreographies by group members. This method is likely to be suitable only for the most competent and creative group participants. At the International Workshop Conference in Melbourne in July 2001 Wolfgang Stange described a choreographic process he has undertaken with intellectually disabled members of his Company Amici. This process requires the group leader to break down choreographic decisions into a stepped process, expressed as questions. In the example Stange described, the participant choreographer's first step was the choice of accompanying music (she chose Vivaldi's 'Four Seasons'). Then, she had to think of her response to a series of artistic decisions such as:

◎   How many people should be in the dance?

◎   When should they start? (altogether? one at a time? in pairs? in a group?)

◎   Which dancer/s should enter the stage first?

◎   From where should they start? (on-stage/off-stage? upstage/downstage? stage right/stage left?)

◎   What should their first step or movement be?

◎   How should they move their body and arms with this first movement?

◎   After the first step, what should they do then?

◎   When they make the second movement, where should they travel to?

◎   And so on.

This chapter has presented a range of issues about performance including various possibilities that are suitable for people with intellectual disabilities, and different models for creating performances. The benefits of performing can include development of leadership and an experience of creative transformation.

The next chapter outlines strategies for successful leadership of groups.

Chapter 7

Strategies for running a group successfully

In the course of running many programs for people with intellectual disabilities, we have developed strategies that help groups function successfully. Not all of these will apply in all circumstances, but setting up a group with them in mind can avoid numerous difficulties. Many of them we learned the hard way. The experience of having a participant going AWOL on the way into or out of a session is a good impetus for the development of more effective strategies for group management!

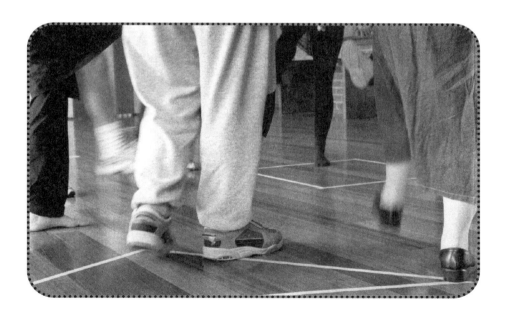

This chapter describes strategies for running a group, beginning with strategies for managing the physical environment. The impact of the external environment on the successful running of a group cannot be underestimated. We then look at issues related to the internal aspects of working with a group, including program management and group dynamics. Finally we look at some of the issues surrounding touch and physical intimacy, and discuss some principles for communicating and facilitating movement.

Managing the physical environment and responsible care of participants

A well set up and organised physical environment will be conducive to the successful functioning of a group following are some suggested strategies.

Working with your community

When a dance program is held in a community setting such as a church hall, it is important that the nature and needs of the group are communicated to other group users and the organising body. The community sharing the venue should have an understanding of the idiosyncrasies of group members so that they do not feel threatened when they come in contact with members. One of the common experiences of outsiders, as well as of new volunteers and staff, is the feeling of being overwhelmed by the unusual behaviours of people with intellectual disabilities. A group leader needs to keep this in mind when supporting people who come in contact with the dance group for the first time.

It can be very useful to talk to other users of the venue about the dance program and its clients, program goals and ways they can support the program. It is also important that the group leader allows time to hear any concerns or questions that individuals or groups may have. On occasions the BreakOut leader has needed to reassure other hall users that sudden outbursts of emotion or odd behaviours are not dangerous, and that staff can deal adequately with the situation. Over time, the community has become familiar and more accepting of the group. They have even offered support to the program in various ways, showing their awareness of the value of BreakOut.

It is also important that other people understand the need for security and privacy of the dance group. At BreakOut we have needed to communicate to other hall users the importance of:

- keeping the exterior door closed
- keeping extraneous noise to a minimum
- keeping the driveway clear so that participants and taxis can arrive and leave safely
- reducing disruptions during class times. As far as possible we request that non-urgent matters are discussed with us outside class time.

There will be times when things happen that are out of the control of the group leader. In a supportive environment, the leader and group are more likely to gain understanding from their hosts. Never forget that a sense of humour is a precious ally in most situations.

Scheduling dance group for uninterrupted time

In the planning stages, a prospective group leader should consult widely with other staff, families and/or carers about the planned program schedule. Avoiding times that conflict with other activities, such as visiting time, morning tea time or weekend sport games, will ensure the least number of disruptions to the dance program.

Choosing an ideal space

The ideal venue is a clear room, large enough to allow for freedom of movement, but not so large as to lose the attention of participants. A carpeted floor is best, so that participants can be encouraged to remove shoes if appropriate.

Having a sprung wooden floor underneath the carpet is very desirable. The concrete slabs on which most modern buildings are set create a safety issue relating to extra pressure on joints from the impact with concrete. If the floor is not flexible, then activities offered must be low-impact, i.e. minimum jumping, bouncing or anything that creates strain on joints and bones.

The ideal room has minimal distractions, though this is something a group leader can control to a degree. Before the session, the group leader should remove objects that may be distracting or dangerous, such as vases and whiteboard markers, to help participants to keep focused. Heavy objects like pianos can be covered or turned around. Exit doors, except the minimum required for safety, should be closed.

An ideal space has a foyer

In programs where one session follows another, the ideal space has an attached foyer, so that people arriving and leaving do not disturb those in the session. If the foyer is set up comfortably with chairs and reading material, parents or carers who are not involved in the class can wait in comfort. This makes their trip to the dance program more pleasant. A separate waiting space can help to ensure that the only people in the dance area are those who are participating, reducing irrelevant conversations, movement and pressure from observers. Participants can prepare themselves for the session by removal of coats, shoes, etc. in an appropriate foyer or waiting area.

Toilet access

The ideal situation is having a toilet close to the dance space, with access from the foyer, thus allowing people arriving and leaving to use it without disturbing the session.

Acoustics

An ideal space is one that is not too large, so music and voices don't need to be very loud to fill it. The best situations are those in which the music and sounds do not disturb those close by, and the sounds made by others do not disturb the group.

Ventilation/heating

An ideal space is flexible in terms of temperature and ventilation. Windows that can be opened and closed are ideal, allowing for plenty of energy-creating oxygen, as is an adjustable heating and cooling system. Body temperature can change within a session, depending on energy expended. The temperature of the environment is best adjusted accordingly, so that there is

- comfortable warmth in the beginning to encourage people to relax, take off their outdoor gear and get involved
- cooler temperature as bodies get warmer from moving
- more warmth at the end during the relaxation/cooldown period, so that participants don't get chilled with the change from vigorous movement to stillness.

Control over lighting

In an ideal situation the leader would have control over the brightness of lighting in the dance space, so that for example, during relaxation time a restful atmosphere could be created by dimming the lights or closing the blinds. This problem can be solved creatively: if there are no dimmers on the lights (highly likely!), lights can be turned off and candles or radiant heaters used as a light source. In one centre where I (Jenny) work, the lights are controlled by key, so I don't have the option of turning them off or down during relaxation. To counter this problem, I provide beanbags for participants to place over their eyes. I am then the only member of the group who has to try and relax under the glare of fluorescent tubes!

Access and supervision issues

The ideal space is easily accessible for wheelchairs, with plenty of parking close by. It is also situated in such a way that participants coming and going can be seen from the dance studio, along with the arrival of parents, carers and taxis. Blinds on windows allow for the outside world to be closed off should it be necessary to improve focus on activities inside the dance space.

Finding the right space for a dance program in a special school

At one special school I (Kim) was allocated the gym as a dance space. This was the obvious choice because it was large and available much of the time. I soon found that the gym was not a good place to work. It was almost always dirty (floor covered in sand from playground equipment coming in and out, so it wasn't comfortable to sit or lie on), cold (mid-winter, and not much heating), acoustically difficult (people found it hard to hear what I was saying), and very exhausting for me. The space was so big that I had to expend a lot of energy holding the class in the space: louder voice, bigger movements, louder music, more space to travel through. When one has to teach all day, one class after another, it is essential to conserve energy to ensure that the last class is as good as the first and that you are strong enough to come back tomorrow and the next day and the next.

I went on a hunt around the school and found a conference room that was carpeted, clean and private. In using it, I did have to make some compromises – like planning for activities that didn't require too much space, re-scheduling my sessions to fit with room availability, and spending time each day moving and replacing furniture. But all of these changes were well worth it for the increased comfort and focus I and my students were able to enjoy.

Dealing with issues outside the dance program

There are days when class plans are best abandoned due to circumstances beyond the control of the group leader. These might be as diverse as very hot weather, a noisy or distracting physical environment or emotional distress. Sometimes when outside distractions are just too overwhelming, it may be most prudent to abandon all hope of running a co-ordinated dance session. In these situations the best thing to do is to value your own flexibility as leader and go with the flow. Lower your expectations and do something very simple and engaging, such as playing some favourite music and having a sing-along, or change modalities altogether and do some visual artwork, like drawing. The group might go for a walk together and give attention to the sights, sounds and textures of a different environment. Or have a cup of tea and a chat, creating interaction of a different kind. Material that could be useful in future dance sessions might present itself, as could new insights into the personality and lives of participants. An example of an unanticipated benefit of a disrupted session appears below.

An unplanned morning of drawing reveals the energy in Philip's dance

One Saturday at BreakOut a working bee was going on in the garden surrounding the hall. As it was a hot morning, we needed both the windows and curtains open to provide ventilation. Despite my attempts to get the morning's dancing started, most participants remained more interested in what was happening outside the building. Knowing that the distractions would continue for the duration of the morning, I (Jenny) decided this was an opportunity for a drawing session with the group. I felt that drawing would be more enjoyable in such hot weather and would provide something concrete for each person to focus on. Fortunately on this day I had butcher paper and crayons in the boot of my car which I was able to access without further disruption to the group. Once settled on the floor, group members were happy to engage in the drawing activity and gradually paid less attention to what was happening outside.

On completion of the drawings, each group member was asked to show and describe what they had done. The descriptions varied in length and content, but most people were able to answer questions directed to them in relation to their drawing. The discussion brought about by the drawing revealed something about each person not previously known or experienced in the context of the dance session. One group member's drawing came as a big surprise. Philip, an autistic man, whose movement is almost always heavy, lethargic and confined, produced a drawing that expressed intensity and energy. He filled a large piece of butcher's paper with strong bright colours in a pattern of intersecting lines and curves. My assistant described Philip's drawing as 'electric'. This activity provided another window into Philip's life for us at BreakOut. We saw him expressing himself in an active energetic way that we don't often see in the dance context. With new awareness of Philip's capacity for expression, I found myself tuned in more to the subtle ways that he expresses his aliveness. I now make a connection between the way his face sometimes radiates with vitality when he is moving and the bold creativity expressed in his drawing.

In finding an alternative activity to do on this particular morning we still managed to spend meaningful time together. Drawing complemented our dance experience and helped us to expand our knowledge of each other.

Accident and injury prevention and management

The dance space should be as safe as possible. Preparation for a sessions may need to include sweeping floors to remove dirt and foreign objects, putting away tables and furniture with sharp edges, or anything that might fall or be dislodged in the case of vigorous activity. Unnecessary furniture should be removed.

Organisations have different protocols regarding reporting of incidents or injuries. A group leader should find out what those protocols are, and what their responsibilities are in the event of an incident. Most disability and government organisations require a formal report to be filed of any incident involving their clients. Reportable incidents might include physical injuries, falls, epileptic seizures, arguments or altercations that result in emotional distress, and violent outbursts that injure or frighten other participants.

For a leader working in an independent setting, it may be advisable to set up an incident recording and reporting system. This is part of running a service that provides responsible care of participants. It is also advisable for the purposes of insurance coverage. Important facts to include in an incident report are name/s of those involved, the date, place and time, witnesses, description of event, description of injuries, and action taken. This report should be confirmed by a second staff member or responsible adult present when it occurred, if possible. That witness should sign the report to indicate that they agree with the information as recorded. Relevant parents or carers should be informed of the event and any action that was taken. In some cases it may also be advisable to obtain that person's signature to verify that they were informed of all relevant details.

First aid

There should always be at least one person present during dance sessions who has up-to-date first aid credentials. A cold icepack should be available for use on minor injuries.

Remember the acronym for injury treatment: RICED (Geeves, 1990)

- ◎ *Rest:* Stop the activity and sit or lie down to rest the injury.
- ◎ *Ice:* Apply ice to injured body part.
- ◎ *Compression:* Compress injury with bandage or similar to reduce blood flow and bruising.
- ◎ *Elevation:* Elevate injured body part to reduce blood flow and pooling, e.g. place leg on cushion on chair.
- ◎ *Diagnosis:* Any injury that is not just a minor strain or bruise should be seen by a doctor.

The group leader should provide information about the incident to parent or carer, and advise them to seek medical treatment as appropriate.

Participant's family and carer contact details should be kept close at hand and a phone should be available at all times.

Coping with asthma

An asthma management plan should be included on the enrolment form (as discussed below) for any participant who has asthma. Staff will then be clear about any course of action they should take, and when outside assistance, i.e. parents/carers, or ambulance should be sought.

What to do if a participant has an asthma attack (adapted from Rimmer, 1998):

- Remove the person from the room and take them to a quiet place.
- Place them in a comfortable position (usually sitting down with the arms placed over a table or chair to help them 'open' up the chest).
- Encourage them to breathe deeply and slowly (diaphragmatic breathing).
- A warm drink may help loosen mucus secretions. Do not give cold drinks as this may cause further tightening of the chest.
- Seek medical attention if symptoms do not improve in a few minutes.

Enrolment procedure

Information needed to provide responsible care of participants might include:

Support and communication
- What kind of support does this person need? How can it be provided in the program?
- What are the drop-off/pick-up arrangements?

Care requirements
- Will a carer attend with the participant?
- Will it be the same carer each time?
- Will the carer be involved in the activity or just be on hand in case of emergency?
- What are the carer's feelings about their attendance/involvement? (see also Chapter 9 on working with a team)
- For non-verbal participants, what are the best strategies for communication with that person?
- What are the person's particular physical/medical limitations or concerns/issues?
- What medical conditions are present?

Emergency plans
- What should program staff do if something goes wrong?
- Emergency contact phone numbers of at least two people
- Doctor's contact number
- Signed permission to seek medical advice in an emergency when none of the listed contact people are available.

Other
- Is there anything else the group leader should know about the participant?

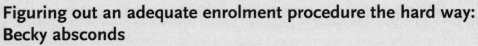

Figuring out an adequate enrolment procedure the hard way: Becky absconds

I (Kim) added this last question about 'anything else we should know' to our enrolment form after an incident in which a participant in a social dance night I was running went missing from the venue. Becky had let herself out of the venue via a locked back door and over a 3-metre cyclone wire fence. She was eventually located wandering the streets of the city at 4 a.m. the next morning.

In discussing with Becky's parents how this very worrying event had occurred, we discovered that she regularly absconded from home and work. They hadn't told us this when they brought Becky to the dance, nor when they filled in the form that requested information about relevant medical conditions.

After hearing of her escapades, we requested that in the future Becky be accompanied to the dance by a carer. We felt that staff running the event were unable to provide the level of supervision that she required. We then began to ask families and carers specifically for 'any other information we should know' about dance attendees, so that we could be pro-active rather than re-active in managing behaviours and providing the safest possible environment.

Insurance

Dance group activities need to be covered by insurance, both professional indemnity and public liability. This coverage should also extend to group staff, volunteers and parents or carers while they are involved in the program. It should also cover group activities when they take place outside the regular venue, for example, a community performance or social outing. Class attendance lists provide a good record of attendance that may be necessary in the unlikely event of insurance claims. A staff/volunteer sign-in book can be useful for a similar purpose.

In Australia, Ausdance can provide contact details for the Safedance scheme that is specifically tailored to the dance industry.

Program management and group dynamics

Creating a friendly atmosphere

An important aspect of a dance program is the opportunity it provides for social interaction between participants, their carers and families. The group leader can foster friendships by creating a conducive environment. Some strategies include:

◉ arriving at class a little early to chat with participants

◉ introducing participants, their families and carers to each other, especially those whose children or clients have something in common (e.g. age, ability, home locality)

◉ providing a foyer space where participants can socialise before or after class, and where parents and carers who are waiting during class can chat in comfort

◉ occasionally holding a social event outside the dance program.

Over time, participants are likely to develop rewarding friendships with others in the group, thereby enhancing their sense of belonging and motivation to attend.

BreakOut trip to Fish Creek

One Saturday when the regular venue for BreakOut was unavailable, we decided to organise a bus trip. The focal point for the day was lunch in a café in a small seaside town. The café was run by Marita Smith, the founder and much-loved former leader of BreakOut.

Catching up with our old friend Marita, followed by a walk on the beach and a rousing sing-along all the way home were highlights of the day. Participants, staff and family members all enjoyed the opportunity to get to know each other outside the usual setting. The enjoyment of the big trip and the shared memory adds to the collection of experiences each member has had as part of the BreakOut group.

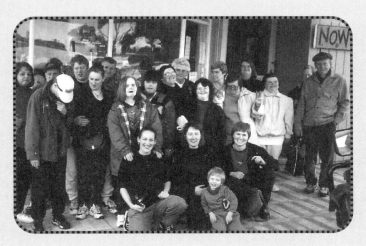

Leadership skills

A group leader's skills can significantly affect participants' enjoyment of the program. It must be clear to participants, carers and families that dance program staff enjoy working with them and are genuinely interested in their wellbeing. Sincere warmth plus the enthusiasm for the dance program will go a long way towards gaining participants' trust and enjoyment. In addition, a successful group leader should also:

- be trained in relevant aspects of dance
- have current first aid training
- have at least a rudimentary knowledge of disability and issues faced by participants
- be able to offer a mixture of fun, purposeful activities
- be able to relate meaningfully to people with intellectual disabilities, their families and carers
- be willing, interested and empathic
- be patient with themselves and others
- be organised in their methods and directions
- be firm but not authoritarian
- be trained in group dynamics (adapted from Lewis and Campanelli 1990).

Group leaders should keep their qualifications up to date and continually strive to improve their professional abilities. More ideas about professional development and networking can be found at the end of Chapter 8.

Communication skills

The following strategies for communication and motivation of participants are adapted from Thompson and Hoekenga (1998).

Step 1: Beginning the session

- Introduce yourself and let participants know that it is time to begin.
- Explain what you will be doing that day and how you expect them to participate. This is especially important when working with new group members.
- Reassure members that they can participate at their own pace, and will not be expected to do things that they are unable or uncomfortable to do.

Concentrate on:

- setting a positive tone ('I'm glad to see you all here today.')
- focusing participants' attention on the class ('Now its time for us to begin our warm-up.')
- explaining what to expect ('After the warm-up today we are going to try some group work using the giant elastic.')
- reviewing prior performance ('Last week, we worked in pairs with smaller elastic. Today we are going to try it with us all working together').

Step 2: Leading the session

Concentrate on:

- providing clear instructions (words first, then physical demonstration)
- giving plenty of genuine, positive feedback ('Craig, you are putting a lot of energy into holding that elastic tightly!')
- actively engaging members' participation ('Does anyone have an idea of a shape we could all make with this elastic?').

Step 3: Closing the session

This sets the tone for the feelings participants carry out of the session, so be sure to close on a positive note.

- Review what has been accomplished and preview what will happen in the next session.
- Summarise participants' achievements ('Everyone has worked really hard today giving their ideas for a new choreography for our concert.')
- Invite participants' comments about their experience of the session. You might ask: 'What movement did you enjoy today?' This feedback can help the group leader understand how the work was perceived by participants and could form a basis for future session planning.
- Express the expectation of seeing them again ('I'll look forward to seeing you next week.').

The more effectively the group leader communicates with class members, the more they will enjoy their participation and the more motivated they will be to keep attending.

The fun factor:

Strategies for making the dance class enjoyable

A group leader can take their work seriously without always taking themselves seriously. Leaders who use humour are perceived to be more likeable and effective. When humour is part of a learning situation, the benefits can include increased motivation, creativity, satisfaction, productivity and decreased stress (Thompson and Hoekenga 1998). Humour assists in gaining and keeping participants' attention and helps everyone to enjoy themselves more. Dean (1993) makes the following points about the use of humour:

- Making fun of oneself from time to time is OK, but making fun of others is not.
- The leader should laugh with others, not at them.
- Show participants that it is OK to laugh. If the leader can relax and laugh from time to time, so will class members.

Tips for handling nervousness or anxiety

Taking on a new challenge can often provoke nerves, even in the most experienced group leader. Some ideas to help control nerves (adapted from Thompson and Hoekenga, 1998):

Before the session

◎   Arrive early for the session, so you can take your time setting up without feeling rushed.

◎   To be sure you feel confident with what you are planning to do, rehearse it in advance.

◎   Visualise yourself as a confident and successful group leader. Picture the best case scenario of how you would like the session to go.

During the session

◎   Focus on the value of what you are teaching and its benefit for participants. This will take the focus off yourself and back on to class members.

◎   Practise empathy: Put yourself in participants' shoes. This helps you teach them better and takes attention away from your own anxiety

Rules about food:

No food/drink/smoking during class-time

This rule may help clients who have difficulty with cravings for food, coffee or sugar, as well as helping you make an arrangement with staff that will work for you. I (Kim) have had the experience of staff in an institution delivering afternoon tea in the middle of my session. This is a sure way to kill participants' motivation to move! If the session is long, set a special time for a snack and a drink. If possible, have a separate space for the consumption of food and drink.

Except for water!

Do however, encourage participants to have small sips of water during vigorous activity or in warm weather. More frequent drinks should be encouraged in very hot weather.

Shoes on or off?

While creative dance teachers often encourage participants to remove their shoes in class, this can be less desirable for some people with disabilities. For people who have structural problems with their feet, like some of those with cerebral palsy, or people with Down syndrome who have hypotonic muscles, support from shoes and/or orthotics makes movement easier and safer. Some organisations have occupational health and safety regulations that necessitate the wearing of shoes, so the group leader should check out those rules before requesting that participants take shoes off.

However, it can be beneficial to encourage class members to take their shoes off during suitable activities. Activities that are not weight-bearing, such as seated stretches and relaxation, can be enjoyable and safe without shoes. The soles of bare feet are very sensitive and are a great spot place for receiving tactile stimulation. The sense of freedom and lightness that can be experienced with bare feet can be a factor that contributes to the transformation of movement from the everyday to the extraordinary.

Sessional group leading: The drawbacks

The sessional nature of dance group leading has its limitations. A leader who spends only an hour or two a week with a group is unlikely to have much awareness of members' wider work and home lives. This can be an advantage, giving participants the freedom to shape a new identity for a new situation. At other times it can be a drawback, when the group leader is unaware of life events that are significant for people in the group.

Strategies that can help a sessional group leader to become more familiar with participants' lives can include:

- Timetabling to allow for a brief catch-up time with parents/carers and participants before or after sessions.
- Having a brief catch-up chat within the session. The group leader might ask participants to share with the class something that happened since the last session.
- Making use of any opportunities to spend some out-of-class time with participants, for example, during the transition between programs, on the walk to the lunchroom after a session, morning tea break.
- Setting up special events such as a trip to a live performance, going out for a meal or something as simple as a morning tea get-together after class or watching a video together.

The story below describes some strategies I (Jenny) have used to create a 'window' into the lives of group members.

Time out for a cuppa and a chat helps group members get to know each other better

One of the groups I (Jenny) worked with met for one hour on a weeknight in a special recreation centre for adults with intellectual disabilities. With only an hour, there was not much time to enjoy a meandering catch-up at the beginning of the session or at the end when some carers and taxis were waiting to take people home. I found the limited time frustrating, as there was never an opportunity to listen attentively to the stories that people wanted to share. One participant, for example, picked a flower on her way to the session each week, and she always wanted to share with me long descriptions of its colour and shape.

I decided that it was important for me to arrive and be set up at least ten minutes before the session, so that I would be available to talk with people as they arrived. Members responded by coming early and sharing with me things about their life: what movie they had been to see, whose birthday they had just celebrated, the excitement of a new found love, the anticipation of a trip home to visit family, sometimes the tragedy of a death. This ten minutes gave me a little window into members' lives that made the experience of dancing together even richer.

continued

During the year we created our own opportunities to celebrate together. At Easter time we had hot-cross buns, in the middle of the year we had a group birthday party to celebrate everyone's birthday, and then there were end-of-year and Christmas celebrations. For these occasions, we would plan a party the week before and people would bring food along to the session. We would begin by dancing together and then set up for our party. Everyone enjoyed this break from the routine. In the relaxed and happy environment of these special events I had the opportunity once again of getting to know my group members better.

One year the centre kindly organised for our group to have our end-of-year celebrations at the local pizza parlour. We all looked forward to this for weeks and people came dressed in their best clothes on the night. However I was really disappointed to find that in the restaurant we were unable to enjoy the same relaxed and chatty atmosphere that we so often had on other occasions at the centre. I wondered if the special room at the centre provided a familiar space in which we could feel at ease and safe with one another? Or if the experience of dancing together prior to eating helped relax the group and create intimacy? The restaurant visit did make me appreciate the relationships we had created together in the dance space. I was reminded of the importance of familiarity when looking for opportunities to deepen friendships.

Touch and physical intimacy: Some issues

Issues to do with appropriateness of touch and sexuality sometimes arise in a dance session. While relationship and sexuality education is beyond the responsibility of a dance group leader, it is essential that the leader is clear about boundaries for staff and class members and

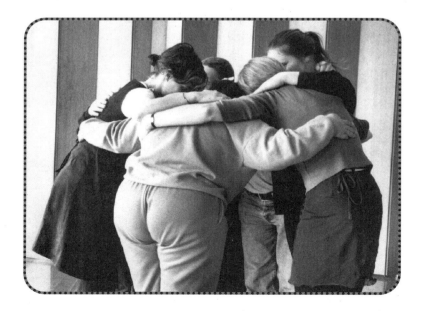

appropriate class behaviour. The dance session may be somewhat challenging for people who have difficulty with those boundaries, especially as touch and physical contact that would be inappropriate in other circumstances may be part of the program. For example, in a dance session acceptable behaviour can include close physical contact between virtual strangers.

A creative dance program can help to educate people about what is 'good' touch, i.e. touch that a participant has given consent to and that is appropriate in the circumstances, given the relationship between the parties and the situation – whether it is a public or private place.

Understanding the difference between 'good' and 'bad' touch can help participants set boundaries for themselves. The experience of 'good' touch that is appropriate and has a clearly defined intention and boundaries can also help participants develop an understanding that touch is not always about sexuality. For example, the pushing/pulling/melting activities described in Chapter 2 require close body contact between partners.

The leader should be specific about what is acceptable in the dance space. Touching of intimate body parts is not, nor is intimate kissing. Participants also need to be encouraged to be clear about their comfort zone and feel free to express concerns or withdraw from an activity or partner if they are uncomfortable.

The same standards of behaviour that would be applied to anyone else in the community should also be applied to people with intellectual disabilities. Group members can be encouraged to shake hands as a greeting unless they are very good friends. A behaviour that makes someone in the dance group feel uncomfortable is likely to have the same effect on people in the wider community. Social skills that are appropriate in the mainstream community should be modelled and reinforced in the dance session.

Issues about body contact surface during a contact improvisation workshop

I (Kim) attended a workshop in contact improvisation with a large group of people, with and without disabilities. At one stage, I began working with a male stranger in an activity that involved full body contact. As the exercise progressed, I became increasingly uncomfortable about the physical relationship with this partner. Eventually I realised that under other circumstances I would not have paired up with a man I did not know for an exercise that required such close contact. Nor would I have continued with the exercise, given my discomfort, if my partner had not had a disability. I decided that my response of discomfort was not unreasonable, and I brought our partnership to a halt. My partner received the feedback that I was uncomfortable working with him in this way. For the rest of the workshop, I chose to pair up with women whenever the activity required close body contact.

A useful schema for discussion about appropriate behaviour is the Circles Concept, designed to help people with intellectual disabilities determine the level of physical intimacy appropriate in different relationships.

Teaching tip: The Circles Concept of Intimacy and Relationships

The Circles Concept is a visually structured approach to clarifying relationship norms and expectations (Champagne and Walker-Hirsch, 1993). The concept explains the range of relationships in which people become involved and the social behaviour that will lead to acceptance by others. The level of physical intimacy appropriate in various relationships is set out as a series of concentric circles, with the appropriate level of physical contact between people defined by their relationship. People who don't know each other, i.e. strangers, generally have no physical contact. People who know each other slightly, like people in the neighbourhood, wave to each other. People who know each other as acquaintances or who are introduced by another person, usually shake hands as a greeting. People who are good friends can hug each other. Only those who are very close and have known each other for some time, like girlfriend and boyfriends, husbands and wives, parents and children can cuddle each other. The innermost circle is oneself and one's own body. Every person has the right to control their own body. They can decide who they want in their innermost circles and how they are to be touched by other people.

If a participant is regularly having difficulty understanding or adhering to behaviour program staff regard as acceptable, carers or parents should be advised. They can seek further training with social skills as appropriate. Seeking further help will ultimately benefit the individual concerned, program staff and group members.

Principles for communicating and facilitating movement

The following section outlines a range of strategies that can assist a group leader to communicate with and facilitate movement of individual clients.

Attunement

Attunement is a technique used by dance therapists to identify with an individual and offer comfort and affirmation of an individual's experience of themselves through

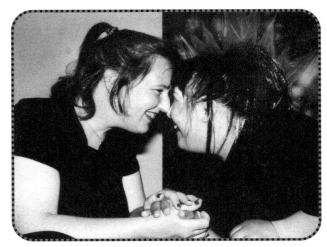

movement. It is the process of the therapist responsively duplicating changes in muscle tension of a mover (Loman and Merman, 1996), and can be considered similar to kinaesthetic empathy. Attunement relies on intuition and is a means of communicating that needs no words. Using attunement to share another person's experience is about creating a safe, permissive and non-judgmental environment. Dance therapists use attunement to 'start where that person is' and establish a deep empathic rapport. This concept is the opposite of the behaviour modification approach that is so much part of the life experience of many people with disabilities. Being attuned to another person is more about getting into their shoes than getting them to change their shoes.

Experience it yourself first

If you ever do something to someone else, make sure you have had the experience yourself first. You cannot imagine how a movement feels when it is done to you, unless you have felt it yourself. Keep in mind also that some of your participants may have vision impairment. If you close your eyes as a movement is done to you, you will experience how movement intensifies when vision is restricted. What do you experience when you were moved quickly as compared to being moved firmly but gently and slowly? The question to ask yourself is, 'Was I able to engage in the movement myself when it was done quickly to me?' If the answer is no, then someone else will be likely to have the same experience. It is important that a participant can engage in movement, even if they cannot initiate it for themselves.

We learned a good lesson about how it feels to be propelled around when we each had a turn in a wheelchair during a vigorous bush dance. Activities we lead for people who need to be manipulated by others have been much slower and calmer since, with much better advance warnings.

Take your time

It is important to work at a speed that is appropriate for class members. As a group leader, you need to be aware of your own movement preferences and the way they impact on your leadership style. If you are a naturally fast mover or talker it will be necessary for you to be very conscious of that fact when you are working with people who need more time. For example, people with neurological disorders and some people with cerebral palsy need to work at a pace slow enough for information to process through the brain and into the body. Otherwise the experience can be one of movement being forced upon a person when they are possibly capable of responding themselves. The experience of learning through movement will be much deeper when an individual is able to process the information and respond independently.

Keep the program routine structured

For some participants, especially those with autism, a structured routine (i.e. same room, same equipment, same music, same group leader) will need to be established. Fundamentally, structure is there to assist participants to feel at ease and give them a sense of security about what is expected. It also gives the group leader a security and familiarity in the process of working with a group.

This doesn't mean that a leader should never vary activities or try something new. It is important to be conscious of structures that are being used and to be aware of when it is important to keep things the same, and when it might be beneficial to vary them in some way, perhaps adding, subtracting or changing.

The time to experiment with change is after a leader and a group have become familiar with each other and have mastered basic principles of dance/movement, such as body control, positioning, relationship with others and space. Participants need to be confident in the current structure before they are ready to be extended into new developments. Structure should be de-constructed so that people have the opportunity to work with independence and freedom. This process should be gradual so that is manageable and changes take place within a familiar format.

Changing familiar class structure leads to surprising outcomes

At BreakOut each person has the opportunity to perform a short solo during the warm-up. Over the years this practice has become a familiar and much-loved start to the session. Each person has developed the confidence to step into the centre of the circle and lead the group with their favourite movement sequence. Sometimes there are variations in members' chosen movements, but mostly this invitation elicits a well-practised response. As the group leader, I (Jenny) have always found the predictability of this ritual very comforting.

One Saturday after the warm-up, I drew a pattern of squares on the floor with masking tape. My intention was that participants would use the squares to direct their movement through space by stepping, jumping or leaping from one square to another. This activity began with participants moving through the squares one at a time, the same way they are invited to share a move in the warm-up circle. One group member, Craig, whose signature movement is a predictable series of strong jumps, surprised us with a Fred Astaire-style tap dance in one of the squares. My assistant and I looked at each other with amazement, as we had never seen Craig move like that before. When Craig first came to BreakOut five years earlier, he sat for many months curled up in a corner. Over the years, he developed confidence to stand in the circle and gradually began to create his own jumping movements when it was his turn to share a move. We have enjoyed watching Craig find his stomp as a movement that expresses his presence in the group. On this Saturday, Craig boldly showed us that he was ready for more than the circle was permitting. He shuffled and wove his feet in and out of the squares with a lightness of movement that contrasted distinctly with his characteristic stomp.

Upon reflection, I (Jenny) realised that the circle warm-up, while providing a comfortable and safe ritual, could also be limiting. Craig showed us that after some years, he was able and confident to move independently of the support provided to him by the circle. I also realised that, although the circle had been removed, the squares provided a means of containing the activity. They were an important transition device between the support of the circle and the challenge of dancing alone in a wide-open space.

Tactile input

Some participants may require tactile input to guide them through a movement sequence, especially if activities are challenging and involve determining or changing directions. A hand gently placed on the shoulder, arm, back or hand of the moving person can help guide them in the right direction. Some people also need tactile input to affirm their physical presence and keep them connected to the group. Use of tactile cues can reduce the number of verbal cues that need to be given and can be a more effective means of communication for people who have difficulty with language. They can also enhance the movement experience by enabling it to flow. Again, sensitivity is vital.

Co-active assistance

Some people, especially those who are less mobile because of a physical disability, may need co-active assistance, i.e. hands-on facilitation of movement by a staff member in consultation with the participant. This allows for a fuller engagement in activities and can make movement easier. If the experience is to be non-intrusive for the participant, a relationship of trust between that person and the staff member is required.

The session could begin by simply touching and talking - for example, saying hello with a handshake or some way of connecting through touch of hands. The person will be able to make a connection between the tactile experience and a voice. Time should be allowed for the person to become familiar with this experience. Once a trusting relationship is established it is then possible to give more direction to movement. Co-active assistance takes time, sensitivity and a willingness to listen.

The following is a description of how an activity could be co-actively facilitated for a participant with severely physical disabilities:

◎ Begin with a prompt such as, 'Christopher, we are going to hold hands and sway to the music.'

◎ Clearly describe the movement, for example, 'I am now placing my hand in your hand'.

◎ Ask for feedback on the experience drawing on the person's individual communication skills, for example, 'Can you hear the music? Can you feel your body swaying?'

◎ Wait for a 'yes' or 'no' response.

◎ Continue the movement slowly before increasing speed or changing rhythm.

Offering encouragement: Verbal and non-verbal strategies

Some group members may need encouragement to participate in a session. Staff need to develop a non-intrusive style of encouragement so that each person has the freedom to participate at their own level. This might mean standing next to a more withdrawn member and making a special effort to say hello. The group leader needs to remember that being part of a group can sometimes be difficult. The assistant is a good person to offer 'one-to-one' support if required in this way. As relationships develop, it will be easier to determine whether the use of touch is a good way of establishing contact. If so, gently holding a person's hand or giving it a friendly squeeze may be welcomed and offers a very personal way of affirming someone's presence.

Participants can also be encouraged simply by hearing their own name, so it is important to begin a session with an activity that uses each person's name. Making eye contact and giving the person an engaging smile when their name is said may be all that is needed to give them the confidence to get involved. All participants will feel that their presence is valued if this is done successfully.

It is also a pleasing experience for a group leader or staff member to be the recipient of similar affirmation. Participants might use eye contact, a welcoming hug, a joke or the sharing of a personal story to express the value they place on your presence. The feeling of being valued in people's lives can contribute enormously to a group leader's sense of meaning in their work.

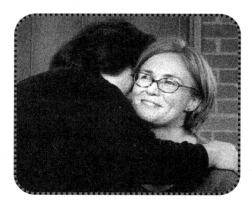

Verbal prompting

There are situations where more directive prompting can be helpful in facilitating a person's involvement. Often children and adults with autism need prompting to help them move beyond their internal world and into a relationship with others. One approach is to encourage them to look at the person leading the movement, who may be the leader or a group member, and offer them a challenge, for example, 'Robbie, can you move your arms like Sarah?' Always use the person's name to begin a prompt and follow it with a clear question or statement.

Sometimes people can wander off and get involved in an activity that is not related to the session. To encourage that person to come back to the group, you can make a statement to remind them what the group is doing, for example, 'Jack we are moving our feet now'. Some people, especially those with autism, may need 'time-out' when demands of group co-operation become overwhelming, and will look for opportunities to leave the group. It is important to acknowledge this need and provide an appropriate space, while also having strategies as described above to encourage focus and participation. Work at phrasing prompts so that they are inviting rather than demanding. Never physically or verbally force anyone to move.

Coping with participants in distress

Sometimes participants come to dance sessions in a distressed state. It can be challenging for a group leader to understand the cause of that distress and to determine whether they have any role to play in alleviating it. This is particularly difficult if the person isn't able to adequately communicate the nature of their worries. Some examples we have encountered include a participant's distress at arriving early or late for the session, anxiety over the unexpected absence of a class member, changing home environments and the recent death of a friend. Strategies we use to deal with distress include offering the opportunity to have a talk about it, either with the group as a whole, or where a second staff member is available, in a one-on-one chat. Changing to a calming activity like those listed in the relaxation section of Chapter 2 can also be helpful. As far as possible, we follow up issues of concern with family members or carers who have a more comprehensive picture of an individual's life. Often they will recommend ideas to facilitate a better relationship with their client or child.

Giving feedback

Types of feedback: Positive, descriptive, negative and corrective

People with intellectual disabilities often have fairly controlled lives and receive a large amount of feedback that is directed at shaping or changing their behaviour. One of the beauties of the Laban model of creative dance is that there is no right or wrong way. Participants have the opportunity to just be themselves and express how they are feeling, without having to be concerned about the rightness or wrongness of it. However, a group leader can use feedback to enhance participants' confidence and motivation.

Positive feedback is a response that tells a person or a group what they are doing well (Hughes, Ginnet and Curphy 1998). An example of positive feedback, is, 'Good co-operation, Sarah and Marc', 'Great jumps, Jana'. The effectiveness of positive feedback can be extended by the addition of description.

Descriptive feedback

Descriptive feedback is when the leader verbally describes what they have observed. For example, 'Fiona, I see how you have stretched out your fingers to the very tips.' When the leader uses descriptive feedback, rather than just a non-specific 'Good' or 'Come on', they are forced to stay fully present in the moment and to be very specific about their observations. In receiving descriptive feedback, the participant is also clear about exactly how they are moving and is affirmed for their efforts and achievements. For example, 'Simon, you are making an interesting shape using your arms and hands', or 'Jenny, I see the way you are using your fingers to make contact with Jon.'

It is also possible to use descriptive feedback as a means of encouraging participants to extend their movements or experiment with new ones. For example, 'Craig, you are stamping with a lot of strong energy today. Now can you find another way to step? Maybe you could try moving without making much sound?' 'Melissa and Tabetha, the two of you together have made an interesting shape. What kind of new shape could you make if you added another person to the group?'

Describing feelings and aesthetic response

A further development of the descriptive feedback process is sharing one's feelings or aesthetic response to an action or movement (Stinson 1988). For example, 'I felt so proud to see the whole group co-operating so well'(feelings), or 'Erica, the flowing movements in your arms made me think of waves in the sea' (aesthetic response). However, the response need not only be positive. For example, 'Doreen, I felt disappointed when you pinched David and disturbed his concentration.'

Feedback from peers

It need not only be staff whose feedback is of value. Taking the feedback process a step further, students can be encouraged to offer feedback to fellow group members after watching an improvised piece or a mini-performance. The group leader must structure this process of giving/receiving feedback in such a way that the student receiving it is encouraged into further achievement, rather than discouraged by comparison or negativity.

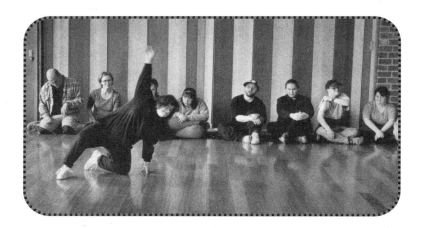

A good starting point for stimulating descriptive feedback responses from group members is the question: 'What did you see?' For some groups, this may be as far as it is feasible to go with verbal questioning. However, if members have good verbal communication skills, they might be asked:

'How did you feel about it? What were the things you liked and why? What could be improved?'

Feedback that comes from peers can be particularly motivating, sometimes more so than the constant voice of the group leader. We have been surprised at how often group leader's views are shared by other class members, thus reducing the need for the group leader to be the one to be always saying 'Come on … join in … reach more … bend more … What else can you do?…'

Jenny's experience with Day Centre group member Delia is a good example of how effective feedback from peers can be.

Delia responds to descriptive feedback

Delia has the shyness of a teenager, though she is in her late twenties. Her shyness is accentuated by her lack of confidence in moving due to her mild cerebral palsy. Locomotion and balance are challenging to Delia. When the focus is turned on her, she will often retreat into a state of contraction and say 'no'. However, Delia loves to dance. During the free dance at the end of the session she can be seen hopping and jumping with joy in the corner of the room.

Over an eight-month period of participation in a creative movement program, Delia developed a movement repertoire that she was prepared to share with the group. Her confidence developed as a result of the feedback from fellow class members. Each session we would have a performance section for participants to perform a solo to their own choice of music. At first, Delia would not perform on her own, so she also chose a partner, and she would only stand still and occasionally hop. When the group was asked what they liked about Delia's dance, one person noticed the hop and told Delia, 'I liked the way you jumped up and down'. This brought a smile to her face.

Delia began to experiment with a quick walk around the room with the occasional hop. Delia's peers had developed good observation skills by this stage, and one of them noticed this progress and told Delia, 'I like the way you use the whole room'. As the group leader, I (Jenny) had modelled ways of giving feedback and encouraged group members to do the same with verbal language. Some people also used non-verbal gestures to indicate their appreciation of a member's performance, for example, thumbs up or thumbs down. As audience members, the group had been encouraged to actively participate by looking for the ways in which the performer's body and the space around them were being used. Group members also seemed to enjoy being asked what they liked and what they saw. The combination of these factors meant that Delia was receiving enthusiastic and descriptive feedback.

After receiving that information, Delia began to move around the room with more confidence, experimenting with speed and using all the space available. She was gradually able to lead her partner in a circle dance of running and hopping around the room and then eventually to perform her 'dance' as a solo. This process showed that Delia was able to direct her own movement. It seemed like a miracle to me!

For Delia, the ability to dance and perform was always there, but she needed to develop her confidence and find movement that she enjoyed doing. The feedback she received from her peers helped her find that. As the group leader, I was able to relax when Delia refused to participate in the warm-up section of the session, knowing that she would be waiting eagerly for her peers' attention and encouragement in the performance section. Through this process I discovered that prompting from me was not an effective way to encourage Delia's participation and enjoyment of dance. Receiving encouraging feedback from her peers was a major factor in Delia becoming able to create and perform her own movements.

Negative and corrective feedback

There may be occasions when non-affirming strategies are appropriate, for example, when a participant is doing something that may be injurious to them, or they have lost concentration or focus or are disrupting other class members.

Negative feedback is a response that tells a person or a group what they are doing wrong (Hughes, Ginnet and Curphy 1998). For example, 'Maria, we are not doing push-ups any more'. Negative feedback is not helpful if participants do not know what else to do, so it should be immediately followed by corrective information. 'Maria, now we are trying to touch our toes!' This can also be useful if a member is distracted or disruptive in a session.

Corrective feedback provides specific instruction on how to improve or extend the activity. It is helpful to supplement corrective feedback by modelling the action you are wanting to encourage. For example, 'See how far I can stretch?', as you model reaching for your toes.

Negative and corrective feedback are most appropriate when the leader is familiar with group and trust has been developed. These can be effective techniques to help expand and develop members' participation and movement repertoire, especially if the leader judges that a member is working below potential. However, a leader's first priority must be to affirm members' sense of self-worth and to value each individual's contribution, whatever it might be.

To ensure that participants stay confident and motivated, it is best to give positive feedback in conjunction with negative and corrective feedback. One way to do this is to use the sandwich technique, i.e. place negative and corrective feedback between two instances of positive feedback (Hughes, Ginnet and Curphy 1998). Start on a positive note and end on a positive note. For example, 'Luke, the first warm-up movement you showed was fun for us all to do. Now you are going so fast we can't keep up with you. I am sure you can think of something we could all do.'

Remember to give positive feedback as soon as participants attempt working in the way you are requesting. To keep them motivated, give positive feedback about each successive step towards the desired outcome in conjunction with corrective instructions. For example: 'That is more like it, Scott. Now see if you can let your head drop even further forward. Great work!'

Improving feedback skills

Hughes, Ginnet and Curphy (1998) suggest a number of tips for improving feedback skills. They suggest that feedback should always:

- be helpful (emphasise behaviours that are under the participant's control)
- be specific (give a clear understanding of what behaviours need to be changed and how to change them)
- be timely (give feedback as soon as possible after the behaviour is observed)
- include positive and corrective feedback. A mix of recognition for what is right, plus ongoing suggestions for improvement can optimise participants' achievements.

Benefits of feedback for the recipient

This process of giving and receiving descriptive feedback can benefit both performers and observers to develop a range of skills. For the performer, possible benefits of receiving descriptive feedback about their movement and dance include:

- increased sense of self as separate and distinct from others

- increased expressive range through heightened awareness of current patterns and limitations, and encouragement to have new movement experiences

- increased ability to make choices with the experience of decision-making through dance performance

- increased confidence with self-presentation in front of an audience with the regular experience of positive learning experiences through performance

- increased enjoyment of performing with regular experience

- increased sense of achievement.

Benefits of feedback for the observer

For the observer, the skills that can be developed through the practice of giving feedback may include:

- heightened observational skills

- increased attentional focus

    (These two skills are particularly useful for group members who have trouble being fully present in a group and tuned in to others.)

- development of verbal skills – through finding words to describe an observation or a feeling.

- development of a vocabulary about movement – words to describe movements such as spin, fly, roll, run slide, jump, slow, quick

- development of a vocabulary around feelings in response to movement observed: 'I felt happy when I was gliding like a kite', 'It was boring when Larry went around and around on the spot', 'It was scary when Erica and Melissa went back to back into the middle and I thought they would crash.'

- aesthetic appreciation: having to make choices about what is aesthetically appealing to oneself and the reason, e.g. 'I liked when Julia went down and spun around on the ground because she seemed so happy'.

There may be members who feel more comfortable or successful giving feedback in movement rather than in words. Contributions of any kind should be encouraged from class members.

Reduce verbal input: Trust in the power of movement

Having said all of that, it is important to keep the amount of verbal encouragement to a minimum, given that an underlying aim in all dance and movement sessions is to communicate non-verbally through the use of the body. With less talk, there is greater focus on the use of the body and being physically present in the movement dynamic of the group. It can be very challenging at first for a group leader to try and reduce verbal input, especially when a group is in its early stages. As rapport with a group develops, the group leader's confidence in leadership and trust in the power of movement to communicate and motivate should make it easier to have less reliance on words.

Chapter **8**

How to set up a dance group and make it work

The professional life of a dance group leader or therapist is not straightforward, easy or lucrative. There are very few full-time positions for such professionals, with no foreseeable change to that situation. However, it is possible to construct a living for yourself in the field of dance and disability, provided that you are entrepreneurial, persistent and hardworking. Below, we describe a range of the ways we have managed to cobble together full-time professional workloads, allowing us to make the most of our expertise and to survive.

We have been involved with a large number of groups, managed in many different ways. The advantages and challenges of each of these situations are described below, allowing a prospective group leader/teacher to judge what situations may be appropriate for themselves depending on their skills, experience and interests.

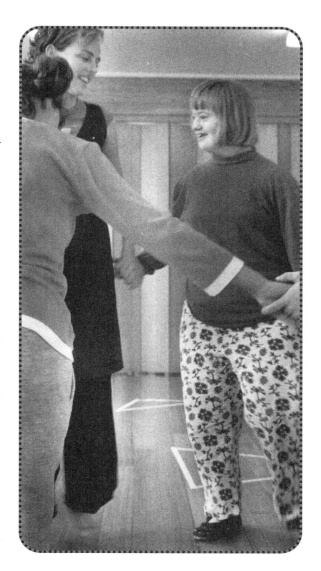

Groups we have led

Community-based: BreakOut Dance Group Incorporated

BreakOut has been set up as a non-profit group separate from any other agency. The original group was supported by disability agency and based in a community dance school venue. Ten years later, the group functions as an independent non-profit incorporated association, offering recreational expressive dance classes to children, young and older adults.

Program focus

Developing creativity, recreation, fun, physical fitness, weekend social activity

Structure	Advantages	Challenges
Autonomous community-based organisation	Independence: no boss, no larger agenda, unlimited scope for change, innovation	No support from larger agency, no structure in which to work
Run by parent–participant committee	All those involved committed to value of dance for participants	Limited input from committee
Incorporated Association	Eligible for community/government grants	Requires regular committee meetings, annual general meeting, annual report, monthly and annual financial report, own insurance. Profits from activities, if any, go to group, not leader
Community-based	Philosophically appropriate for recreational activity	Can be lonely and isolating for staff.
Participants are self-selected and pay their own way	Participants motivated and interested in activity	No guarantee of participants / income
Hire own staff and select volunteers	Support staff can be selected for their skill/expertise in dance/disability and shared vision	Limited pool of appropriately skilled staff. Staff wages have to come out of class income
Organise own venue	Can control venue (size, availability, cleanliness, set-up, heating, etc)	Have to finance the hire of venue from income
		Responsible for hire contract, payment

Community Centre-based: Act It Out program

These weekly dance/drama sessions are held for clients (an adults/older adults group and a young adults group) in a local council-funded community centre. Some clients come independently from the community, paying for these sessions themselves. Others attend with their day program groups and are paid for with the funding their centres receive from the state government to run the day program.

Program focus

Communication skills development, expressive, performance focus

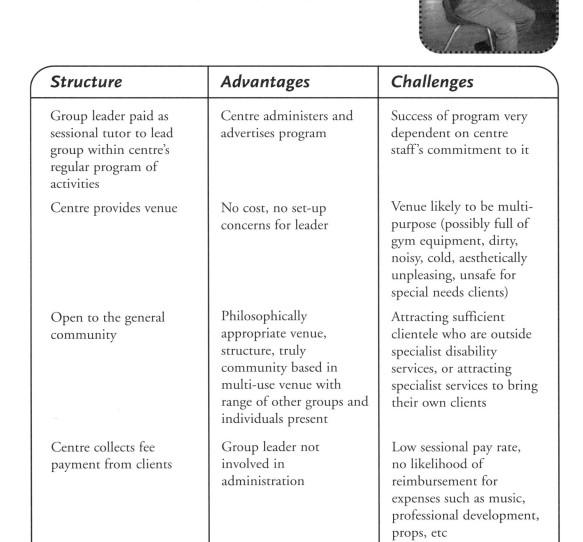

Structure	Advantages	Challenges
Group leader paid as sessional tutor to lead group within centre's regular program of activities	Centre administers and advertises program	Success of program very dependent on centre staff's commitment to it
Centre provides venue	No cost, no set-up concerns for leader	Venue likely to be multi-purpose (possibly full of gym equipment, dirty, noisy, cold, aesthetically unpleasing, unsafe for special needs clients)
Open to the general community	Philosophically appropriate venue, structure, truly community based in multi-use venue with range of other groups and individuals present	Attracting sufficient clientele who are outside specialist disability services, or attracting specialist services to bring their own clients
Centre collects fee payment from clients	Group leader not involved in administration	Low sessional pay rate, no likelihood of reimbursement for expenses such as music, professional development, props, etc
Centre insures group	No insurance issues for group leader	None

Community Centre-based creative arts program: Avalon Centre Incorporated

Avalon is a non-profit organisation that aims to provide creative opportunities for people who are disadvantaged (physically, mentally, intellectually, socially or emotionally). Jenny was impressed by the centre's philosophy and made contact with the co-ordinator, Deborah Holmes, a drama therapist. The two decided to combine their skills in a 'creative arts day', offering drama and dance as a full-day program. This idea was then marketed to a number of Adult Training and Support Services (ATSS), with the outcome of two centres combining to bring 14 clients to Avalon for the day.

Program focus

Social interaction, creative expression, personal development, improved body and spatial awareness.

Structure	Advantages	Challenges
A day program offered to ATSS and other disability support services outside their centre	The centre's aim is to provide creative opportunities for people who are disadvantaged. No need to convince the organisation that this is a good idea	A lot of travelling is involved for clients. Once they have arrived at their day centre they then travel again. Programs can be cut short in order to juggle transport logistics
	The team works with a drama therapist. Programs can be developed to complement each other	Range of age and needs can vary considerably within the one group
Venue provided by centre and in keeping with the centre's philosophy	Not institutional. Offers a homely environment away from the client's regular day centres. Relaxed, private and functional	Not a purpose-built venue. Limited space for working with large groups
The disability service pays for the 'creative arts day'. Avalon then pays for the dance program from this money	Marketing/advertising provided by the centre. Group leader not involved in administration	Group leader has limited involvement in the bigger picture, e.g. program funding can be cut without consultation. Clients can withdraw from program without opportunity for a follow up
Support workers attend with clients	Support workers have more information about participants lives outside dance program	High turn over of support workers

Recreational program based in a residential service: The Oakleigh Centre

This weekly session came about after the recreation manager at a large residential centre for people with intellectual disabilities was sent a brochure about BreakOut. After discussion about financial and transport issues, it seemed most pragmatic for the BreakOut leader to attend the centre and run an in-house session for residential clients. The client group has now expanded to include community members – non-centre clients – who live locally.

Program focus

Recreational activity, fun, fitness, creative expression

Structure	Advantages	Challenges
Participant self-select this as a recreational activity and pay for it themselves	Participants are motivated and interested in activity	Program reaches only those clients who enjoy physical activity – those residents who most need physical exercise not likely to attend
Centre's recreation manager administers collection of payments and pays group leader collectively	Financial management easy – Centre's staff ensure enough participants attend to cover minimum fee for group leader	Group leader must be a registered business and invoice for fees
Centre provides venue	Group leader not responsible for maintenance, open up/lock up of building, not required to organise contract, payment of rent. Fees relatively cheap for participants because fewer costs and risk for group leader. Activity takes place in a building with other activities going on – not too lonely	Not truly community based: specialised setting. Group leader has little control over venue, cleanliness, space available, suitability
Centre provides some resources, e.g. CD player	Group leader may not have to lug heavy equipment	CD player may not be ideal for dance class purposes

Agency-based: Brimbank Disability Support Service

Brimbank is a day activity centre that services young adults with mild and moderate intellectual disabilities. The centre offers creative arts activities to complement skill-based programs. Clients have the opportunity to be involved in music, drama, art and dance, as well as travel training, cooking, gardening, computer skills, etc. People who need to increase their participation in physical activity, or improve co-ordination, self-confidence and positive social interaction are recommended to participate in the dance program. The program exists because the centre values the role of creativity in the social, emotional and physical development of their clients. Jenny has worked at the centre one day a week in a permanent capacity.

Program focus

Developing social skills, creative expression, personal development (self-esteem and confidence), increased mobility

Structure	Advantages	Challenges
Creative movement is part of the centre's regular program	Program is valued by the centre. Dance group leader is valued as a specialist Working as a team member and being part of the bigger picture	Keeping up to date with developments in the centre and with clients. Staff meetings are held outside dance group leader's paid working hours
Clients are recommended to participate in the program to help them achieve their individual goals for social, emotional and physical development	Clients are respected as individuals and the program aims to support their needs	It is difficult to follow through client's interest in dance outside the centre
Support workers available according to the needs of the group	Skilled and informed support staff available	Funding changes can affect the number of support workers available High turnover of support workers means time and training needed to create rapport
Program funded by the governing body (charity and council)	The program can receive extra funding to cater for special needs Regular income for group leader A full day's work in one centre	Dance group leader paid as a casual employee and therefore not paid when centre is closed
Purpose built venue	Insurance can be covered by the centre	

Day activity and training centres: Various programs

During a period of employment as a regional community worker with the state government disability services, I (Kim) was able to spend some of my paid time using my specialist expertise in dance to offer programs that enhanced choices for clients attending day programs at these centres. The range of possibilities this included were:

◎   lunchtime jazz–fitness programs, attended mostly by young adult female clients

◎   a series of folkdance classes leading up to a concert presentation for more able children

◎   one-to-one therapeutic dance sessions for individual high-need clients.

Program focus

Recreational, physical fitness, skills development – performance, skills development – therapeutic

Structure	Advantages	Challenges
Day Centre programs – group leader's time funded indirectly by state government. Low demand workload of official duties allows some time to be spent on area of interest to group leader, thereby extending the range of regular programs that centres could offer clients	No financial issues for clients or centre.	The ongoing nature of these programs requires a continued low-demand workload of official duties, and implicit, if not explicit, agreement of employer (i.e. state government management)
Centre provides venue	No cost, no set-up issues for group leader	Not community-based. Venue likely to be multi-purpose (possibly full of gym equipment, dirty, noisy, cold, aesthetically unpleasing, unsafe for special needs clients)
Centre provides participants by encouraging current clientele to participate	Easily accessible clients, who may really enjoy and appreciate new opportunity at no cost	Requires centre staff to be appropriately supportive of value of dance and clients' participation, providing program time and venue and support staff

Hospital-based: Music and movement sessions for geriatric patients with intellectual disabilities - Brierly Hospital, Warrnambool

This program came about when a social worker at a psycho-geriatric hospital realised that some clients who had been institutionalised for most of their lives had amassed large sums of money from their pension funds. They had no access to these funds and nothing to spend them on. The social worker began a campaign to set up some activities that would enhance the quality of life for those clients, financed by their own savings. One of these was a music and movement program.

Program focus
Physical exercise, therapeutic movement, social interaction, intellectual stimulation

Structure	*Advantages*	*Challenges*
Hospital-based	Easily accessible clients, desperately in need of exercise, stimulation, new ideas and input	Hospital staff make decisions about who attends, clients not necessarily capable of making or expressing informed choices. Not all staff supportive of program, large bureaucracy to deal with for any changes, innovation, issues
Venue provided	Sessions affordable to participants as no rental fee necessary	Hospital venue appropriate for clients for age and support needs of clients. Group leader has no control over space, what other activities go on in there at the same time, cleanliness, volume of other activities
Support staff available in hospital	No need to hire outside staff, therefore cheaper for clients, easier for group leader	Hospital staff not necessarily motivated, or interested in being involved, no continuity of staff. Staff accustomed to doing things 'to' clients, rather than with them, counter to dance therapist perspective/intention of stimulating client to do things themselves
Clients pay for session from pensions, these collected and disbursed to group leader by hospital administration	Financial aspect easy for group leader	Only those with sufficient funds able to attend

Special school artist-in-residence program: Bayside Special Developmental School

This residence was set up at a special developmental school after an approach by me (Kim) to the principal of the school, suggesting that we apply together for funding from the state government's 'Artists in Schools Scheme'. The success of this funding application meant that I was able run a weekly full-day program for 20 weeks, involving most students in the school. The focal point of the residency was the creation of a performance for the Combined Special Schools' Music Festival.

Program focus

Artistic, educational, performance outcome

Structure	Advantages	Challenges
Special school hosts an 'Artist in Residence' for limited period	School enthusiastic about new program that is not part of regular curriculum Raises profile and reputation of school in the community	Artist does not 'belong' to school Limited involvement can mean limited impact on students and staff
School staff act as assistants	Artist has the opportunity to be involved with teachers and introduce them to new ideas re possibilities for dance and movement activities for their students. No cost involved, staff have specialist disability training	Staff may not be enthusiastic about dance program, no specialist skills in dance
Outside agency, e.g. state government arts/education department, funds program	During period of funding round, no financial issues for school or artist	Artist and school have to write a successful funding submission for a program that has a limited life
School provides venue	No cost, no set up concerns for artist, usually safe and special needs student-proof venue, no insurance required by artist	Venue likely to be multi-purpose (possibly full of gym equipment, dirty, noisy, cold, aesthetically unpleasing)

Early intervention program for children with special needs: Noah's Ark Family Resource Centre

I (Kim) was involved with a movement and music program for children with special needs at non-government agency early intervention service. This program had been running successfully for some time, led by a dance therapist and assistant with training in early intervention, supported by graduate dance education students. I began as a volunteer on graduate student placement and worked for some time in that capacity, before running the program myself for a time.

Program focus
Early intervention, educational, social, parent–child relationship building

Structure	Advantages	Challenges
Weekly sessions for mothers and preschoolers with special needs in an early intervention centre	Centre mostly philosophically in tune with idea of movement as modality for development	Occasional challenges from therapists from other disciplines regarding relative value of dance program
Parents paid little or nothing to attend. Centre's activities mostly covered by state government funding	Group leader not involved in financial management. Low-income families not prohibited from attending	Ongoing nature of program dependent on state government funding and commitment of centre management to program
Centre provides support staff, from other disciplines including early intervention, physio and occupational therapy specialists	Support staff generally specialists in disability area – dance group leader works as part of a team Excellent resource for parents with access to staff from various disciplines	Possibility of challenge to leadership from support staff member with expertise outside group leader's range

Other possibilities for program structure

There are yet other possible ways dance–movement groups can be set up for people with disabilities. These might include:

◎ sponsoring/hosting by a disability agency, e.g. the Down Syndrome Association

◎ after-school activity at a special school

◎ private tuition arranged by parents

◎ special-needs classes in a mainstream dance school

◎ integrated group suitable for high-functioning clients.

◎ participation in mainstream dance programs. That is perhaps the ideal and is entirely possible for high-functioning people with appropriate support.

Techniques for survival as a dance group leader

Support group and supervision: Set yourself up in a network

One of the most important things to do as a dance group leader is to develop a support network for yourself. You need to be in contact with others who share your belief in the value of dance, who are having similar experiences so you can talk through problems with them, who can support you – perhaps even lead your group when you are sick or when you are having a break, and who can help you on performance days.

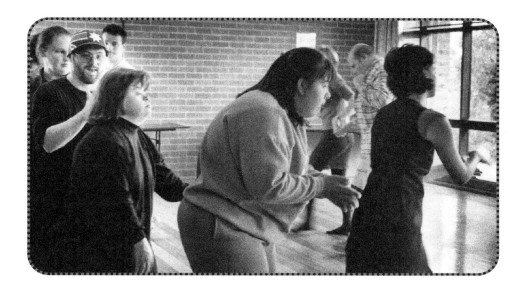

Ideas for building a network

◉ Join your local dance organisation for example: Ausdance in Australia or the National Dance Association in the US and get involved in the area that relates to your interests.

◉ Join the Dance Therapy Association (DTAA in Australia, ADTA in the United States) in your state. If there isn't a branch close by, get one going.

◉ Join any disability advisory groups that your local council may run. Disability agency workers will get to know you and your group, and be more inclined to refer clients to you, and you will have an extra support with disability specialists.

◉ Join disability associations that are relevant, e.g. The Down Syndrome Association, Autism Australia, VICSRAPID (Victorian Association for Sport and Recreation for People with Intellectual Disabilities).

◉ Inform institutions who are training potential assistants or teachers about your group (universities, TAFE colleges, specialist training organisations such as IDTIA – International Dance Therapy Training Institute of Australia). You will then be likely to attract volunteers – students on placement, new graduates or people in career transition who can offer you assistance while they learn.

Keep up your professional skills

It is essential that you keep your professional skills up-to-date and stay on the lookout for new and enlivening experiences to draw upon. Keep reading about other people's work, thinking, talking and writing about your own, and attending training programs and workshops. Continual development of your skills means that you will do a better job at what you do, and also allows for the possibility of change and development in your professional life. There may come a time in the future when a change of career focus becomes desirable or necessary, and the more training and skills you have, the more likely you are to be able to meet those different requirements.

Some areas to consider in your professional development include:

◉ first aid and injury management

◉ occupational health and safety issues, such as safe manual lifting techniques

◉ small business management/legal issues, perhaps offered by organisations such as Arts Management Advisory Group

◉ disability relevant training: e.g. communication skills, behavioural management techniques, policy and philosophical issues around disability practice

◉ dance education theory and practice

◉ dance therapy theory and practice

◉ other dance styles and techniques, such as folk or social dance, improvisation

◉ complementary creative arts, drama, music, visual art, etc.

◉ complementary body therapies such as Pilates, yoga, Feldenkrais, massage

Succession: The importance of training students and volunteers

Offering hands-on training opportunities in your program to students and volunteers will contribute significantly to its long-term success. People new to the field are usually very enthusiastic and energetic, and can provide a good complement to the more experienced and possibly more worn-out leader.

The ideal training model would be for a prospective group leader to undertake formal professional training while doing a placement or volunteer work with an experienced leader. If a prospective volunteer is not in professional training, a group leader might encourage them to investigate appropriate courses.

To complement formal education, a group leader can offer invaluable on-the-job training which might include:

- some involvement in program planning, at least enough to understand the process
- an opportunity to see and experience appropriate techniques for group management being modelled by a skilled and experienced leader
- graduated opportunities for leadership, as discussed in Chapter 9.
- regular feedback/discussion with other staff members after a session
- appropriate reading material. The group leader might recommend or lend references to the student on disability, dance therapy, Laban creative dance, etc. (We have written this book for those students!)
- suggesting/inviting the students to join professional organisations or networks (as listed on previous page)
- referral to other groups for complementary training, e.g. other disability arts programs, groups that work with other disability issues, such as people with physical disabilities, groups working with age or ability levels that are different from those in your program
- information about professional development opportunities and if possible, funding for fees.

When a new staff member is needed for a program, a person who has already been working with the group will be an obvious choice. When the group leader wants to move on from a particular job or organisation, someone who is already experienced with that group will then possibly be in a position to take over. This succession model means less disruption for program participants and an easier transition for staff members who are leaving or taking over. A program will be more likely to have continued success if it is left with a well-trained leader.

Marketing your program and your skills

If you want to earn money every week(!), you will need to continually market yourself and your program. The more people and agencies who know of you and your work, the more participants and opportunities will come your way.

These are some of the strategies that we have found to be effective:

- Enlist participants, carers and families to assist with the task of promoting the program. Word of mouth is always the best publicity.

◎ Use your program to promote itself. Outward-focused activities, such as community performances, special events involving invited guests and audience, 'invite a friend' day all help to raise consciousness of your group's activities.

◎ Make a brochure about your program that includes your training and experience, and send it regularly to relevant agencies, such as early intervention centres, special schools, day centres, residential agencies, disability support agencies (e.g. Down Syndrome Association, Yooralla, Autism Australia) and arts agencies (including Arts Access, peak bodies such as Ausdance), local councils arts, recreation and disability programs, community and arts centres. Address it personally to staff to whom you think your program might be relevant, e.g. the recreation officer, physical education teacher, respite care co-ordinator.

◎ As far as possible, make personal contact with people who might refer clients or groups to you. Having met you, they are much more likely to have faith in you and your work. Making yourself known within these networks will make it more likely that:
  ● projects
  ● participants
  ● job opportunities/contracts
  ● students/volunteers
  ● funding
  ● staff
  ● performing opportunities will flow towards you.

◎ Join relevant professional organisations and
  ● get to know your peers in the field
  ● receive their newsletters
  ● attend meetings.

◎ Become involved in promoting the field of disability arts as a whole. You will become more informed, better at what you do and more likely to find appropriate staff, volunteers, funding, support and venues.

◎ Attend conferences, talk about your work and learn about what others are doing.

◎ Use the media – local and specialised. For example, get an article and a photo of your group in the local paper. You will be more successful at this process if you have an angle that sounds interesting to journalists – an upcoming performance, for example.

◎ Write an article for a professional journal. Jenny, was who living in London, found her way to BreakOut in Melbourne, as a result of reading an article in the Dance Therapy Association of Australia Journal. Think local and informal about this, e.g. your local arts network monthly broadsheet, or national and international, like the Journal of Intellectual and Developmental Disability or the American Journal on Mental Retardation.

These strategies offer a way of exploring the potential for working in and further developing the field of dance and disability.

Chapter **9**

Creating a successful team

It is important for a dance group leader to have positive relationships with program staff, other colleagues and those who are involved on the periphery of the dance program, such as parents, carers, support staff and managers. The establishment of good co-operation between all parties can be assisted by clear delineation of roles and responsibilities. To follow are some ideas for clarifying expectations that we have developed in the course of managing numerous groups.

The role of an assistant

The assistant helps to keep the magic in the moment by reducing distractions. A supportive assistant is often the key to running a cohesive and dynamic program that has minimal disruptions.

When a group enters fully into the dance experience, a type of magic is created. Keeping this magic requires the group leader to be fully attuned to the dynamics of the group and the individuality of each member, and to be able to respond creatively to these through movement. This magic can easily be broken by distractions, so it is helpful to have strategies in place to diffuse their impact. An environment free from interruptions will enable group members to be more creative and express more of their individuality.

Preparation for a session should include a discussion between the group leader and the assistant about issues that might arise and appropriate responses. These might include management tasks such as setting up the space, supervising the arrival and departure of participants, noting absentees, collecting money, distributing notices, ventilation/heating control, and how to handle health and behavioural concerns such as injuries and emotional outbursts. Clarification of the assistant's role means that s/he can attend to these tasks without further discussion during the session.

Agreeing on teaching and feedback strategies

Before a new assistant starts work, it is advisable for the group leader to discuss with them how interaction with participants will be best managed during the session. Decide in advance who should do the talking, and how support can be provided for participants without taking away from the focus of the session. Should the leader do the talking and the assistant play a more silent, supportive role? Clarifying this ahead of time saves awkwardness later.

Creating a dynamic of play together

Playful interaction between group leader and assistant can be an effective way of getting a group started. This can be especially useful for groups who are difficult to engage, like the older adults group at BreakOut. These participants have few verbal communication and limited social interactive skills, and often take quite a long time to become involved in any kind of group activity. When a playful dynamic is set up between the group leader and the assistant there is usually a response from class members. This response stimulates engagement, and with engagement comes the beginning of movement dialogue. The willingness of the assistant to enter into play can be one of the group's best assets in difficult situations.

Assistant and group leader create a dynamic that involves reluctant participants

It was one of those mornings when establishing focus in the group was proving difficult. The warm-up exercise did not inspire participation and group members were distracted by activities outside the dance space. Abandoning my plan for the session, I (Jenny) began by rolling a very large ball into the middle of the circle. I then rolled it towards our assistant, Karina, who picked up the ball and balanced it on her head. This drew the attention from outside the room to the inside, as it became more interesting to see what would happen to the ball than what was happening in the car park. Karina let the ball roll from her head and bounce across the circle, where it stopped in front of my feet. I then picked up the ball and, pretending that it was very heavy, walked around the circle looking for someone who would take it from me. The ball had now become the focus of the group. Karina took it from me and placed it in front of group member Judy's feet. Judy was very excited to have control of the ball and yelled 'wow' as she kicked it across the room. Before long everyone in the circle was kicking the ball. The group had come alive!

Providing emotional support for participants

Providing individualised emotional support to participants is a key role of an assistant. Participants may come to a session distressed about events in their lives, or be overwhelmed by an emotion during the program. The group may need to stop whatever they are doing to create space for such a response. If a brief break does not address the member's need, the assistant can take some time out of class with them to talk, walk or share a cup of tea. Time-out is often a good way to diffuse the impact upon the group and still give an individual the attention and care they need.

Quiet time provides an opportunity for emotional support for Georgia

Georgia, a member of the young adults group at BreakOut, sometimes became very upset when a particular friend did not turn up to class, and she would burst into tears and run out of the room. We discovered that the best remedy for Georgia in this situation was to have some one-to-one time with the assistant to share her feelings over a cup of tea. We suspected that Georgia's distress over the absence of this group member had some connection with her experiences of loss and abandonment as a child, as when she got upset, Georgia would talk about her foster family and how far away they were and how much she was wanting to see them. It seemed to help if she received some intimate support and reassurance from the assistant. After some quiet time, Georgia would come back to the group happy to join in activities.

Georgia has gradually become more able to cope with changes as they occur in the group. However, her need for emotional security is a reminder that routine and familiarity are very important in creating an environment where all group members feel safe.

Providing emotional support for the group leader

The assistant can also provide emotional support to the group leader when the two work as a team. It is wonderful to feel the support of an assistant on those days when your spirits are low or you just cannot find the energy to meet the group. Sharing the challenges can halve the burden, and together difficulties become surmountable.

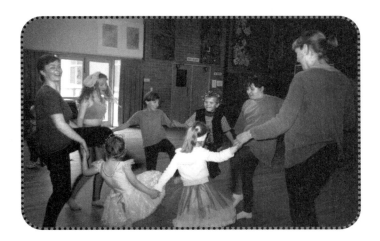

It is equally special to share the breakthroughs: those moments when someone makes eye contact for the first time or moves spontaneously into the centre of a circle, when previously they have not engaged. Savouring achievements together can affirm your sense of the worth of your work.

Reviewing the session together

It is important to make time at the end of the session to review what took place. The leader needs to create time for the assistant to give feedback on what they experienced within themselves, for example, 'Today I had lots of energy and I was very excited to be here,' or 'I found today hard and I feel exhausted,' while also sharing the leader's own experiences. The two can then spend some time discussing observations of each group member's participation and reviewing aspects of the session that could have worked better. When a review is carried out together, the leader is acknowledging the assistant's important contribution to the program, as well as creating a discussion that can lead to growth and change for staff and the group.

Training: Graduated experiences for leadership

An assistant can develop confidence to lead the group through graduated opportunities for leadership. This process can begin with the assistant directing one section of the session. The warm-up at the beginning or relaxation at the end are ideal because they can have such clear structure and intentions. Sharing leadership roles with the assistant could be a regular pattern or something that is discussed and planned prior to the session. Stepping into the role of leader is a different experience for an assistant and requires some preparation.

It is vital that participants are clear about who is leading the session at any particular time, as clear leadership helps maintain focus. When the leader hands over charge of the group to the assistant it is therefore important to say, for example, 'Karina will be leading the warm up today. Can we listen to what Karina would like us to do?' It is then important for the leader to step back and allow the assistant the space to lead. Any comments or suggestions should be kept until review time at the end of the session. The leader should step into the role of assisting and give the group leader their full support.

When the assistant has developed some confidence leading the group, the leader can take the opportunity to step out of the group and observe. There are likely to be aspects of the group's functioning or individual member's responses that become apparent when the group is observed from a less active position. Also, taking some time out on a busy day can help the leader renew energy and focus.

The sharing of leadership roles with an assistant can extend into other activities, such as choreographing a performance piece. If an assistant can accomplish this they have developed both skills and confidence. An assistant who has the confidence to lead is a great asset, as a replacement for the leader when necessary. A person who is familiar with the group and the structure of the session makes the best substitute.

Co-operating with professionals from other disciplines

There can be a lack of congruence between the medical model that deals with people and bodies in a functional way and that of a dance therapist or teacher which focuses on people's capacity for expressive and thoughtful movement experiences. This incongruence can lead to conflict of views about activities that are appropriate for clients between dance group leader/therapists and nursing or other staff.

It is important to establish common ground with other professionals and to have a shared understanding of the purpose of an individual's participation in a dance program. Goal-setting and evaluation issues discussed in Chapter 10 deal with this issue in more depth. One way to do this is to attend an individual's case management meetings and staff meetings. Learning about the objectives of other programs, and sharing those of the dance program, informs you as a dance group leader and other staff members. Any opportunity to share one's knowledge of the value of dance and its role in promoting health and wellbeing should be taken up. Involvement with professionals from other disciplines also assists the dance group leader to extend their own knowledge and understanding of relevant areas. For example, I (Kim) learned about the concept of motor planning for the first time when I worked with a dance therapist who had a background in physiotherapy.

The challenges of working with nursing staff

I (Kim) had my first experience of running a dance program in a hospital when I was fairly young and inexperienced. This was a ward for people with intellectual disabilities who lived long-term as patients in a psycho-geriatric hospital. The challenges there were enormous, particularly as they were associated with entrenched hospital culture of what seemed to me only fairly rudimentary physical care and the relative newness of the idea of recreation activities for patients, especially dance. These activities were unpopular with many staff because they added to the workload, (e.g. having to bring people out from their bedrooms and reorganise furniture) without any obvious benefit to hospital functioning. Clients who had spent most of their lives in institutions were accustomed to spending their days sitting unoccupied in chairs, therefore causing little 'trouble' to staff, and requiring no more than physical care.

Often nursing staff would use my presence as a group leader to take a shared break. While I would be in the loungeroom struggling with a group of up to 20 older adults with high support needs, staff would be laughing together in the tearoom. For me, however, this isolation was often preferable to the presence of staff who were unenthusiastic or even antagonistic about the dance session. Occasionally a staff member who was obviously uncomfortable or unenthusiastic would be rostered on to

continued

work with my group. Sometimes a staff member would get halfway through an activity and then leave to attend to other patients without me knowing if they would return.

At other times a staff member would be assigned to the session, and I would spend energy 'training' them to assist me. Then the hospital roster would rotate and I might have another assistant, who would have to be trained all over again, or there would be no assistance. When I left this job the person who replaced me arranged to have a regular assistant who was not on the hospital staff. Needless to say, she fared much better than I in the job!

Working with families and carers

In dance groups run in community settings, parents and carers can be important team members. Communication between the group leader and these groups is vital to ensure that all parties are clear about the intention of the program, and to enlist the co-operation and support of all. At BreakOut, a number of strategies for achieving communication and co-operation with families/carers have been developed, including:

◎ newsletters/noticeboards: A regular newsletter is created to go home with participants, keeping all involved up-to-date with class activities, coming events and welcoming new participants and staff. This newsletter, along with information from other relevant services, photos of group members and past events, is kept on display on a noticeboard in the foyer of the hall.

◎ committee meetings: BreakOut is run by a management committee that meets once per term. This allows the more enthusiastic participants, carers or parents to have input into management of the group.

◎ performance opportunities: These include informal Open Days for friends and families, where class activities and participants' achievements for the term are highlighted: e.g. an annual performance held in a theatre.

◎ special workshops, perhaps with guest artists, that are open to visitors

◎ outings, such as visits to performances and community events as spectators and /or participants.

The advantages of better communication with families/carers include contribution of ideas for improving interaction with group members.

Given that those who are closest to an individual are usually very skilled at communicating with them, it is prudent for a group leader to be aware of and build on that expertise. Tried and true strategies are a good starting point for communication with a new group member. That is not to say that unexpected responses don't happen. Someone who is not co-operative at home may not necessarily be so in a dance group, especially if they have come to the program willingly.

Johnny's mum helps with communication

Johnny is an eight-year-old boy with autism, who loves to sing, dance and clap out rhythms. His mother, Sandra, was keen for him to try out a class with BreakOut in the hope that it would provide him with a fun, creative and social activity. At the first class, Sandra explained that we needed to be very clear in our communication with Johnny to help him understand what was required of him. She suggested that we begin communication by using his name and simply describing what we wanted him to do. After watching us do the warm-up circle, in which we made movements with different body parts, Sandra suggested that we prompt and encourage Johnny by giving simple instructions such as 'Johnny, hands' or 'Johnny, feet'. I (Jenny) was reluctant to be so directive and I felt confident that eventually Johnny would follow if he was given time, yet I wanted also to be respectful of Sandra's knowledge of her son. I decided to compromise my approach to accommodate her suggestion. Each time I introduced something new, I would prompt Johnny by saying 'Johnny, run' or 'Johnny, jump". After the initial instruction, I would also give him the opportunity to follow the group without further directions. However, I did notice that Johnny still needed prompting to remain engaged in an activity, even after the initial instruction. I was then thankful for Sandra's suggestion and put it into practice by standing beside Johnny and quietly prompting him through the stages of each activity.

This form of direct prompting helped Johnny to become familiar with and successful at the activities of the dance program. After six months, he was very comfortable with the group, as demonstrated by the way he entered the dance class singing, smiling and joining the circle without any hesitation. As Johnny became more relaxed, it was evident that he had the capacity to initiate movement without any prompting. However, whenever when we experiment with a new step, or if Johnny has a day when he is less connected to the group, I use his mother's advice and gently prompt him to re-engage.

Shared understanding of expectations for participants

If parents/carers and dance group staff have shared goals about the purpose of participation in the dance program, there is likely to be more satisfaction. One of the ways to do this is to begin the process of participation in a dance program with a discussion about the person and their family's or carers' motivations for involving them. Why do they come along? What are they hoping to achieve? The group leader can measure those intentions against the likely outcomes of participation in the program and decide if the ideas are commensurate. This strategy is also discussed at length in Chapter 10.

Different expectations of group leader and parent cause embarrassment

Twelve-year-old Karen, who had autism, was a member of the children's group at BreakOut. Karen often found it difficult to co-operate in group activities, especially if they were lengthy, or required intense concentration. We tried hard to create an environment in which it would be easy for her to stay engaged by removing as much irrelevant stimulation from the room as possible. When she reached her capacity for group participation, Karen would often break away from the activity and go off running or skipping around the room, wrapping herself in the fabric of the curtains or mats, or engaging with objects, touching, twirling, twisting. We struggled with decisions about our strategies to deal with Karen, alternating between feeling like it was OK to allow her the quiet time that she obviously needed, and feeling lax for allowing her to indulge in autistic behaviours that were inappropriate in a group setting. I justified her lapses in participation to myself by thinking that, as Karen attended a mainstream school and probably spent all her weekdays struggling to be attentive and co-operative in a group environment, BreakOut might function as an enjoyable contrast and release.

I had never discussed with Karen's mother, Despina, this decision about management of Karen in class. This failure caused embarrassment for me, Karen and her mum, the day Despina came to concert dress rehearsal and found Karen running around the hall on her own while the rest of the group were in a circle focusing on warming up together. I had made the judgment that Karen probably felt overloaded with the stress of being in a new place with a larger group than normal and would be best served by some 'quiet time'. Despina did not share this view, however, and spoke very harshly to Karen about her lack of contribution to the group. I was embarrassed that a conflict between Karen and her mum had arisen as a result of a perhaps inappropriate judgment I had made. I resolved to try and avoid similar situations in future by discussing with all new parents/carers and participants their motivation for coming to class and what they were wanting to achieve. As I got to know participants and new issues arose, I would make a practice of broaching concerns with families/carers, so I could develop a strategy that would fit with their idea of appropriate management. I felt this was the best way to avoid embarrassment, disappointment and family conflicts, and also to share my view of the client/child and my vision for their development through dance.

Benefit for families

Sometimes a dance program can provide a new and positive outlet for an individual. We have found that parents and carers can often be pleasantly surprised to see their child or client participating enthusiastically and expressing themselves creatively in the dance group. This may help them focus on the abilities, rather than the disabilities of people in their care.

Benefits for the group

It can be advantageous for the group to have a pool of involved people to draw on for events that require extra assistance. This could be having someone who can act as an extra driver for a special event, or specialist expertise, perhaps with lighting for a performance or financial management for the committee.

Disadvantages of involvement from parents and carers

There are some drawbacks in having more involvement from carers and parents. The greater the engagement of a carer/parent, the less the group belongs to the participant alone. It is important that the dance class be an independent experience for the person with the disability, and an opportunity for them to express themselves without history of diagnosis or family patterns of relationships.

When a carer's presence can be more a hindrance than a help

Seven-year-old Lachlan was accompanied by a paid carer, Ross, when he joined the junior group at BreakOut. The first week Ross was very willing to participate in the dance session as well, and Lachlan enjoyed having Ross dancing alongside him. The following week, however, Ross wanted to sit out and watch the session, so that Lachlan could participate independently. We supported this decision as our aim for all the children is for them to eventually work independently of parents and carers. Lachlan appeared very at ease with the separation and participated wholeheartedly in all the group's activities.

However, Ross was obviously not as comfortable with the separation process, as became evident when he started to direct Lachlan's activities from the side. Every time I (Jenny) gave a direction to the group, Ross would then repeat the same instructions to Lachlan. When Lachlan completed an activity, Ross would congratulate him with comments such as, 'Well done, Lachlan, that was fantastic'. I found it very distracting to have this extra voice intruding upon the session and it also seemed to disturb Lachlan's focus. While I value positive feedback, I keep it to a minimum, so that the children experience their own sense of reward through the joy of movement. My preference is for descriptive feedback that helps children make a connection between the movement they have made and their achievements, like the following comment, 'Lachlan, you really made me feel excited when you jumped so high'.

As I tried to ignore Ross's verbal intrusions, I hoped that eventually he would become aware of the methods I was using and realise that his instructions were redundant and annoying. However this did not happen. I decided that I needed to explain to him the reasons for my choice of strategies and suggested that Lachlan could be left in my care for the duration of the dance session. With the agreement of Lachlan's mother, Ross's role was reduced to bringing Lachlan to class and collecting him afterwards. This

continued

seemed a much more satisfactory arrangement for all parties. Ross explained that he had felt obliged to keep focused and actively involved in the dance class in order to justify the payment he received as Lachlan's carer for the morning.

This experience with Lachlan's carer taught me the importance of communicating clearly my expectations of parents and carers when they first attend the dance class. While I felt very challenged by this experience at the time, it did prompt me to realise the importance of having strategies to protect the group process and to ensure that children enjoy dance class independent of carers' supervision. Since then, I have been much more direct with parents and carers, explaining that they are welcome to stay with their child for as long as the child needs them and that during this time it is preferable that they actively participate. I specifically request that they do not give their child any feedback until the end of the session, so that the child only has one set of adult instructions to attend to. I encourage them to leave the children with us in the class as soon as they are comfortable to do so.

Managing volunteers

Volunteers can be a welcome bonus or a vital element of a support-intensive program. The group must benefit in some way by the presence of a volunteer, and the volunteer must meet their own needs if they are to make a regular commitment.

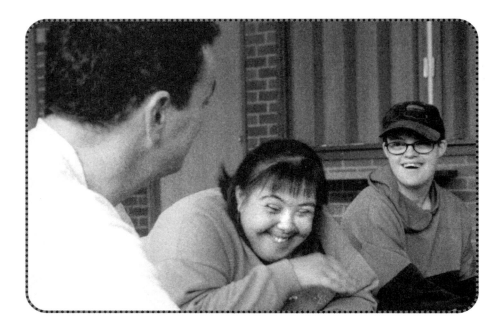

Qualities required in a volunteer

- ◎ maturity (ability to take responsibility for self as well as helping others)
- ◎ willingness to participate in creative activities
- ◎ co-operation
- ◎ reliability, punctuality and consistency
- ◎ respectfulness of group members, other staff, families and carers.

In some cases, where a volunteer is likely to work unsupervised with group members, obtaining a police check may be an advisable preliminary step.

Preliminary discussions are essential to ensure that volunteers' needs are likely to be met by participation in the program and that their skills will benefit the group. Issues that should be clarified include:

- ◎ Are there particular skills that person is wanting to develop by being there?
- ◎ What opportunities are there for them to develop those skills in the dance program?
- ◎ What role do they want to take: a quiet background support role or the opportunity to gain experience as a leader in a supported environment?
- ◎ Are they looking for related employment opportunities? If so, how could the group leader assist with this search?

Occasionally a group may be disrupted or disadvantaged by the presence of a volunteer who needs a lot of support or instruction. A group that is comprised of people with intellectual disabilities is unlikely to accommodate a volunteer whose presence does not contribute more than it costs (in terms of time, energy, support or guidance). An option in this situation might be for the leader to suggest more appropriate volunteer opportunities or give them a referral to a volunteer agency.

The leader should encourage volunteers to develop their skills outside the program by being a positive and inspiring role model as leader, providing information and, where possible, support for training and education, and providing or referring the volunteer to relevant reading material.

Chapter *10*

Program planning and evaluation

Planning a dance program: Establishing goals

The first step in developing a dance program is to clarify the goals to be achieved. This can assure prospective program hosts (for example, managers of day centres or principals of special schools) that a dance program will offer their clients or students experiences that are appropriate for their developmental goals. It will also ensure that activities appropriate for particular clients are offered in a new program. Clear goals will also be useful to assist with the ongoing planning and focus of an established program, especially when participants are ready to move to another level, and can help to re-assure group leaders of the value of their work during the low times.

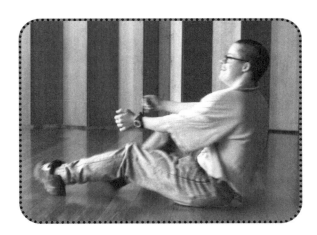

Meeting the goals of all stakeholders

A dance program must meet the goals of a number of stakeholders if it is to have long-term success and viability. By stakeholders we mean people who have an investment in the success of the program. These may include:

- prospective participants and their families/carers
- current participants and their families/carers
- host organisations (i.e. school, day programs for people with disabilities, community centre)
- funding bodies (e.g. Department of Education, Human Services, disability service providers)
- program staff (leader and assistants)

- professional colleagues
- management level decision-makers
- policy-makers.

Different goals may apply to the same program because of the different perspectives of these various stakeholders, as will be discussed below. A competent and effective group leader will need to consider all of these perspectives when planning and evaluating a dance program and will also need to take a pro-active role in advocating the value of the program, and of movement and dance generally.

Prospective participants

A program needs to be attractive and appropriate to potential participants and their parents/carers if it is to be viable in the long term. It must be accessible, affordable, enjoyable and welcoming. As well, programs catering to a particular target group need to be appropriate for the special interests and needs of that group. For example, a program offered to teenagers needs to be up-tempo, fun and 'cool', while a program that caters for older adults needs to be safe, enjoyable and not overly demanding.

Meeting the needs of current participants

The most important stakeholders are current participants. The group leader should clearly understand the motivation of each individual attending the program. Motivations might include enjoyment of dancing, making new friends, hearing favourite music or getting some exercise. Having a participant (if possible), carer or parents establish what an individual's goals are and spelling them out in writing can help a leader to offer a program that is appropriate for that person. This process can also be a way of determining whether the expectations of an individual are likely to be met by a particular program or whether another option might be more appropriate.

Meeting the goals of families/carers

Parents and carers often have an important role in facilitating the attendance of participants, and must therefore be convinced of the unique value of the dance program. The cost of attending (financial, time, energy, inconvenience) must be outweighed by the perceived value of the program to themselves and their child/client. It must also be considered more worthwhile than other similar possibilities, such as other recreational activities. It is therefore important that the goals of families and carers for their client's/child's participation are achieved. These goals might be as diverse as an enjoyable weekend recreational activity, a chance to make new friends, physical exercise or a creative outlet. They may also include personal benefits for the parent or carer, for example, allowing them to have an hour on a Saturday morning to themselves or presenting opportunities for the parent/carer to meet other parents with children with intellectual disabilities.

For parents and carers to have a long-term commitment to the program, the leader needs to offer some interpretation of each individual's challenges and achievements. This can be accomplished through:

- in the case of a children's program a display of lesson plans on a noticeboard near the dance space, outlining activities and their underlying aims and objectives

- for families and carers of non-verbal adults a communication strategy such as a communication book. This level of communication would only be possible in a program of reasonable length (at least half or full day)

- newsletters describing the group's activities for parents/carers who don't come to class

- periodic 'open days', when parents and carers can observe their child's/clients' progress and the group leader can explain dance/movement activities in depth, and the achievements and challenges for class members in undertaking them

- resources, such as reference articles and books available for loan, to those who want to extend their understanding of the field of movement and dance.

I realise that parents need more interpretation of activities to understand their value

I (Kim) began to be much more pro-active in describing the work I was doing in a creative dance program for young children with special needs after two incidents with parents. On both occasions the parents were participating in programs with their children and I had assumed that the purpose and value of the activities were obvious. On the first occasion a parent asked me when the group would begin to 'really dance, and not just run around?' The second occasion was during a relaxation activity where I and the parents were giving 'magic carpet rides' to the children who lay on blankets that we dragged around the floor of the dance space. One mother called out across the room, 'What's the point of this?'

I was surprised at this question, as to me the benefits of the activity were obvious. They included the deep sense of relaxation that all children achieved while 'riding', a moment for each parent and child pair to focus on the special bond between them, the clear sense of individual self and body boundary the child achieved through the firm wrap of the blanket and solid contact with the floor, and above all else, the sheer pleasure of the activity for all; the uplifting music (Brahms 'Lullaby'), a quiet moment in the busy lives of parents and young children, the captivating innocence and beauty of the children lying so tranquilly, and the sense of a shared purpose and love for all the children from the parents and leaders.

When I explained my intentions, the mother was quite surprised at the layers of meaning that I perceived. I hoped that on reflection she would be able to come to an understanding of those things. I resolved that in future I would be more deliberate about describing the purpose of activities we undertook.

Meeting the objectives of the host organisation

The objective of the host organisation must be met for a dance program to have ongoing support. Again, these goals may be different in diverse settings. For example, a community centre that hosts a creative dance program may have set up the program because of funding requirements that they offer weekend recreational activities for people with disabilities. A school may have a commitment to offering creative arts activities to its students as part of its charter. A residential service for people with intellectual disabilities may be aware of the need to offer its clients activities that involve physical exercise. A group leader should be clear what those goals are and ensure that program activities match them.

Mismatch of leader's skills and host organisation's goals spells end of program

A dance/drama program in a special school had been running successfully for some time. It came to a quick end, however, after a program leader who was leaving unwittingly found a replacement for herself in someone whose skills did not match the (hitherto unspoken) goals of the school. The original leader had skills in both dance and drama, and the program she ran drew on both of those art forms, including work on language and creative vocal self-expression. The replacement leader had no drama background and focused the program much more on non-verbal activities.

Neither of these two were aware of the mismatch until the liaison teacher from the special school expressed her discontent with the program content under the second leader. For this teacher, the aspects of the original program that had been most valuable for her students were those that involved verbal expression. She had been happy to have dance content as a complement to the drama aspect of the program but no longer felt convinced of the value of the program when it changed to include predominantly non-verbal activities. This teacher decided to end the program once it no longer matched her goals for her students and no suitable replacement teacher could be found.

Meeting the requirements of funding bodies

Funding bodies almost always have conditions attached to their grants, which must be met. These conditions may be as simple as providing the requisite number of student contact hours per dollar of funding, for example, in an adult education program, while arts bodies are likely to require a successful performance outcome. Funding bodies are also likely to require the satisfactory completion of a written evaluation or report.

A group leader needs to be realistic in terms of likely outcomes when planning and setting up a performance-focused program, especially if they and/or the group are new to the experience of movement and dance. It may be that goals that are appropriate in one context are unreasonable in another.

Meeting the needs of program staff: Leader and assistant/s

Three aspects of the involvement of program staff must be considered.

- the group leader and staff's enjoyment of the program is an important factor in its success, as a group led by people who are not fully committed to the work is unlikely to meet its potential
- the group leader and staff should feel positive about their suitability for their work and the adequacy of their skills and training for the program
- staff need to feel confident about the achievements of themselves and their participants in the program.

Ensuring the value of the dance program in the eyes of other professionals

It is essential that the program has credibility in the eyes of other professionals. These may include colleagues and support workers whose co-operation is needed for the program to work, staff of agencies who may or do refer participants to the program, people who make decisions about funding and support, for example, the committee of a community centre, the school council or policy-makers. These people need to believe that:

- dance is a valuable learning mode,
- the leader and the leader's approach are suitable for the group,
- the desired outcomes are likely to be achieved and
- the outcomes achieved are worthwhile for their clients.

A range of strategies for educating other professionals are outlined below. For those who have immediate contact with the program, professional development activities in which they learn more about the value of the movement and dance experiences are important. These can include:

- informal conversations about the progress and participation of group members in the dance program
- experiential workshops in which other staff undertake the activities themselves. This is one of the most effective ways of understanding the challenges and pleasures of a moving experience
- formal lectures or talks where the program goals and potential outcomes are described by the group leader. This may also include discussion of the way dance activities can function as adjunctive therapies or skill-building programs, for example, how dance may complement the aims of carers working with clients to develop social skills, or physiotherapists working on motor skills.
- theoretical and evaluative references (like this book) that clearly indicate the conceptual underpinning of a program, its value for participants and a sense of a bigger picture, i.e that the field of movement and dance has a history and theory beyond this particular program.

How to make this happen

A dance specialist who is a part-time contractor is unlikely to have much say over the decision-making of an organisation, for example, with regard to the content of professional development activities. It is quite likely that s/he does not attend staff meetings or other events when staff are informed about issues that may be relevant to the dance program, such as updates and reviews of clients, strategies shared by other staff and organisational policy. However, some ideas that have helped us be more effective in organisations include:

◎ offering to lead a workshop for staff

◎ talking about the program's goals and the intention of each activity to support staff while they are working in the dance program, as part of the hands-on training

◎ finding an ally in the organisation, and enlisting their support. This is ideally someone who understands the value of the program and has power in decision-making

◎ familiarising ourselves with the language of the organisation and the model within which the staff are working, then finding a way for the dance program to be aligned with that model, or at least, not be contradictory

◎ undertaking disability training similar to that of other staff to ensure shared understandings.

Advocacy with professionals, funding bodies and others outside the immediate contact zone of the program

It is important to advocate and promote the value of a dance and movement program to people who do not have immediate contact with it such as local, state and federal government, funding bodies and health authorities. Effective advocacy includes three essential components – documentation of programs, evaluation of program outcomes, and dissemination of that evaluation.

Evaluation is not widely used in the arts, but many other professions are making it a priority. Guthrie (2000), for example, discusses the concept of evidence-based therapy used in medicine and health sciences that is essential in the dance and physiotherapy based program she runs in a hospital. In the setting of evidence-based health services it is important to use a model that has proven efficacy and a means of measuring that efficacy after application. This theme of evaluation of dance programs will be expanded in the last section of this chapter.

Planning a dance program: Setting goals for individuals

Learning more about the special needs of particular conditions and disabilities of potential participants can contribute to an appropriate choice of activities in program planning. Particularly useful references include Dykens, Hodapp and Finucane (2000), *Genetics and Mental Retardation Syndromes*, and for a reference that is specifically about children, Batshaw (2002), *Children with Disabilities*. There are several other titles listed in the bibliography. Important questions such as those about participants' physical health concerns and behavioural challenges that need to be part of the enrolment procedure have been discussed in Chapter 2. These all impact on the choice of suitable activities.

Having obtained information about a participant's disability and any psychological or physical concerns, a group leader then needs to be clear about the participant's motivation for coming to the group. This information should be considered when classes are planned. Following are some questions that could be asked.

Ascertaining motivation: Why is a prospective participant choosing this program?

◉ How did the participant find the program? Did someone refer them?

◉ Why was the participant referred to the program?

◉ What is the participant's intention in coming to the program? What do they want to achieve?

◉ Are these intentions shared by carers and families?

◉ If not, what other ideas do parents/carers have?

◉ What does the participant and parents/carers expect of the leader, the program staff and the program?

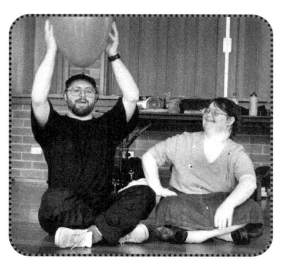

Suitable goals and activities for dance programs

Table 10.1 outlines a whole range of possibilities of goals, activities and intended outcomes for dance/movement groups for people with intellectual disabilities. The choice of goals for a particular group will depend on variables such as the skill and ability level of participants and the purpose of the program. Suitability of the various types of activities for specific populations is also indicated.

The goals in Table 10.1 are listed according to the level of challenge they are likely to present for participants and the populations for whom they are suitable. The list begins with the most basic and essential goal – the creation of a sense of fun and enjoyment. This is a fundamental starting point for all other possible activities.

Table 10.1 GOALS AND ACTIVITIES SUITABLE FOR DANCE PROGRAMS FOR PEOPLE WITH INTELLECTUAL DISABILITIES

Population for whom this is suitable	Goals — What is the purpose of the program?	Actions — What action will be taken to achieve this?	Outcomes — What is the intended outcome of the activity?
All levels of ability	A sense of fun and enjoyment	Group leader creates a relaxed environment Group leader demonstrates a lively sense of humour Program is responsive to unexpected events and responses Program offers opportunities for experimentation with a variety of mediums such as props, songs, music and musical instruments.	An enjoyable experience for its own sake Reduced tension and frustration Group bonding and togetherness Trust and risk-taking Self-expression

continued

All levels of ability	Creating a sense of community Individual feels connected to group as a valued member	Regular ongoing program Organisational stability Group leader creates positive role model through leadership Contribution of the individual to the group is valued Group work, especially improvisation Development of the ability to work within a group to listen, observe and give feedback	Sense of belonging Opportunities for participants to be both recipients and contributors
All levels of ability	Development of the ability to relax	Relaxation exercises including: ◎ body massage ◎ breathing exercises ◎ listening to music ◎ guided meditation	Reduction in body tension Deep, regular breathing Improved focus and body attunement Relaxation as a life skill
Participants with high support needs	Better connection with the here and now	Focusing exercises: ◎ blowing bubbles ◎ passing balloons and balls ◎ singing songs using names ◎ a movement circle group following the movement of a designated leader	Awareness of self, others and the environment
Participants with high support needs	Stronger connection with others	Sharing props, e.g. holding ends of fabric, ribbons or elastics Acknowledging other group members through name games and choosing partners. Duets and small group exercises and improvisations Creating group sculptures	Increased awareness of others Improved relationships to peers and others Connection with others Trust

continued

Population for whom this is suitable	Goals What is the purpose of the program?	Actions What action will be taken to achieve this?	Outcomes What is the intended outcome of the activity?
Participants who are independent* and motivated	Improved body awareness and movement mastery, expansion of movement range	Laban-based movement activities focusing on the use of ⑥ different body parts ⑥ body and space ⑥ effort qualities ⑥ body and relationship (with other people or objects)	Improved awareness of personal space for self and others. Greater skills and confidence in functional movement Greater enjoyment of expressive movement
Participants who are independent and motivated	Enhanced communication skills	Opportunities to use movement to communicate ideas, feelings and emotions Using verbal or sign language to describe movement Using observation skills to develop focus and attentiveness	Increased vocabulary, especially in the use of movement-related words Increased non-verbal communication skills Increased level of attentiveness and interaction Greater self-confidence through richer communication
Participants who are independent and motivated	Improved fitness and co-ordination	Aerobic activity that: ⑥ increases heart rate ⑥ improves balance ⑥ improves co-ordination ⑥ stretches and strengthens muscles	Improved fitness Increased awareness of the importance of fitness for personal health Improved confidence and enjoyment in physical abilities Release of energy

continued

*In this context, independent means individuals who are capable of initiating movement, have cognitive skills to process basic information and are able to work co-operatively in a group.

Participants who are independent and motivated	Improved connection between thought, imagination and body	Activities that encourage the expression of ideas, e.g. sharing personal news, discussing favourite films, creating an imaginary scenario Leader-facilitated exploration of movement and dance Self-initiated exploration of ideas through movement Extending movement experiences through other artforms such as drawing, drama, music-making Performance, observation and feedback	The ability to transcend the everyday A greater awareness of self and skills for self expression Increased creativity and self-empowerment Political challenge to ideas that intellectually disabled people are not creative thinkers
Participants who are independent and motivated	Development of initiative, decision making and leadership skills	Opportunities for participants to make choices in relation to: ◉ initiating activities ◉ leading activities ◉ props	Improved self confidence and assertiveness Greater awareness of personal preferences Taking responsibility as a group member by contributing ideas and helping to make decisions
Confident, independent performers with a strong personal interest in and talent for dance	Performing skills	Regular class participation to develop movement repertoire and confidence in physical expression Rehearsing a repertoire, so that the group develops cohesion, synchronicity and familiarity Creating opportunity to perform in front of an audience ◉ in class ◉ for an invited audience ◉ for a public event	Personal transformation Socially valued role as a performer Contribution to artform of dance Providing enjoyable artistic experience for audiences

This table of goals can be used to structure programs for different populations. Table 10.2 includes examples of program goals selected from Table 10.1 that are appropriate to the needs of three different populations (participants with high support needs, groups that include people with a range of abilities, and highly motivated and independent functioning participants).

Table 10.2	SELECTED GOALS SUITABLE FOR SPECIFIC POPULATIONS
	Bolded words indicate main area of focus with each group.

Population	Program goals
high-support needs participants	**Sense of fun and enjoyment** **Connection with here and now** **Connection with others** **Body awareness** Communication skills Ability to relax
Groups that include people with a range of abilities	Sense of fun and enjoyment Connection with here and now **Connection with others** **Body awareness** **Communication skills** **Fitness and co-ordination** **The ability to relax** **Develop initiative, decision-making and leadership skills** Connection between thought, imagination and body
Highly-motivated and independent functioning participants	Sense of fun and enjoyment Connection with here and now Connection with others Body awareness Communication skills Fitness and co-ordination The ability to relax **Development of initiative, decision-making and leadership skills** **Connection between thought, imagination and body** **Performing skills**

Assessment and evaluation

Why evaluate?

While the primary focus of a creative process such as dance is about the creation of an enjoyable and expressive experience, there are some contexts in which assessment or evaluation are important. In order for stakeholders (such as program hosts or funding bodies) to know whether their goals are being achieved, it is important that the outcomes of participation in a dance program are understood and documented. In dance programs, this process of evaluation is often only done informally, perhaps by the group leader's intuitive sense of what is working, as recorded in session notes.

Other approaches to evaluation and assessment

Interest in the area of evaluation of arts programs is increasing. Writers from fields including community arts, dance therapy and dance are developing, testing and documenting various models. VicHealth has recently sponsored the publication of a tool for evaluating community arts projects (Keating, 2002). While this is not specifically related to dance, it provides a very comprehensive approach to the evaluation processes and outcomes of community-based arts projects. Mead (1999) also discusses evaluation of community-based dance programs and provides a set of simple strategies for undertaking quantitative and qualitative evaluation.

In the area of arts therapy, Feder and Feder (1998) have explored fundamentals and principles that apply to all evaluation; quantitative and qualitative. Their book, *The Art and Science of Evaluation in Arts Therapies* covers specific approaches to evaluation: psychometric, clinical and intuitive. Feder and Feder describe the five functions of evaluation as:

- to ascertain the problems and needs of a person (patient/client or staff member)
- to predict future behaviour
- to monitor change
- to know when to stop
- to learn how to improve treatment methods or techniques (1998, p. 5).

Dance therapists, especially those working in medical settings, are becoming more conscious of issues to do with evaluation and assessment, and are developing tools to that end. The Kestenberg Movement Profile (KMP) is one such tool, well-known in the dance therapy field because it 'broadens and enriches the dance/movement therapist's repertoire of skills for observation and intervention', (Loman and Merman, 1996, p. 29). However, Hill comments on problems with the KMP, in that 'although many dance therapists use [it], there do seem to be difficulties with reliability and inter-observer agreement and dance therapists often seek other tests to combine with the KMP' (2000, p. 3).

Dance therapist and physiotherapist Jane Guthrie comments that 'establishing initial baselines (starting points by assessment), evaluating throughout therapy and documenting the 'outcome' or finishing point should be a standard procedure in any therapy' (2000, p. 4). She applies simple goal setting and measurement of functional outcomes for her clients with acquired brain injury using a range of tools that include Laban Movement Analysis (LMA). Owen, too, uses LMA concepts to assess progress in dance therapy programs. Her (1999) article details the movement observation scale she created for her work with a young man with autism.

Sally Fitt's (1980) 'Simplified Movement Behaviour Analysis' for programs for people with disabilities also draws on LMA principles. This very basic tool for measurement of movement utilises the group leader's observations of participants' movement on scales of Laban's effort qualities of time, space and force (weight). It is very much focused on measuring the mastery of basic movement skills. Fitt gives very detailed descriptions of methods of observing, assessing and quantifying movement behaviour. This reference would be useful for professionals wanting to develop observation skills.

However none of these tools address all of the aspects of a dance program that we have discussed, i.e. development of movement skills as well as creative expression, social interaction, physical fitness and community involvement. Nor were they specifically designed for populations with intellectual disabilities. Therefore, we felt it appropriate to create a simple tool that would be suitable for the evaluation of Laban-based movement and dance programs for people with intellectual disabilities. This tool, which appears as Table 10.3, comprises evaluation strategies for all outcomes listed earlier (in Table 10.1) as suitable for such dance programs.

Table 10.3 ASSESSMENT/EVALUATION TOOL
Refer back to Table 10.1 for the population for whom these goals are suitable.

Goals	How to measure this goal	Scale
A sense of fun and enjoyment	Informal reports from parents and carers	antipathy → enjoyment
	Informal feedback in class	antipathy → enjoyment
	Surveys	antipathy → enjoyment
	Observation of non-verbal behaviour: (facial expression, body stance, relationship)	displeasure → smiling
		tension → ease
		distress (withdrawal, crying, emotional outburst, physical agitation e.g. flapping, rocking, masturbation, dangerous or self-harming behaviour) → playfulness
	Observation of verbal/vocalisations	verbally non-communicative (silent, withdrawn) → communicative (laughing, talking, spontaneous comments)
	Attendance record	infrequent → regular attendance
	Level of involvement	low → high level of involvement
	Level of enthusiasm	apathy → high level of enthusiasm

Goals	How to measure this goal	Scale
Connection with the here and now	Focus on group activity	distracted, (physically restless, scattered attention, inward focus) → focused energy
	Energy attuned appropriately to the activity	clashing → attuned energy (see glossary)
Connection and communication with others	**_Non-verbal communication_**	
	Energy attuned appropriately to partner or group	clashing → attuned energy
	Eye contact	inappropriate → appropriate
	Use of personal space	inappropriate → appropriate
	Initiation of contact	unsuccessful → successful
	Sustainment of contact	unsuccessful → successful
	Release of contact	unsuccessful → successful
	Turn-taking	unsuccessful → successful
	Appropriate physical contact	inappropriate → appropriate
	Verbal communication	
	Expressive verbal interaction	inexpressive → expressive
	Appropriate verbal interaction	inappropriate → appropriate
	Listening, turn-taking, empathising	inappropriate → appropriate
	Confidence in self-expression (verbal and non-verbal)	unconfident → confident expression of personal feelings and experiences
Body awareness, mastery and expansion of movement range	Articulation of body parts	
	Upper: (head, shoulders, arms, hands)	low → high level of articulation
	Centre: (abdominals, chest, pelvis, spine)	low → high level of articulation
	Lower: (legs, knees, ankles, feet)	low → high level of articulation
	Extremities: (arms, wrist, fingers)	low → high level of articulation
	Spatial access: (near, mid, reach, far)	restricted → expansive use of space
	Access to effort qualities:	
	⊚ flow (bound – free)	low → high level of access
	⊚ space (direct – indirect)	low → high level of access
	⊚ weight (light – strong)	low → high level of access
	⊚ time (sustained – sudden)	low → high level of access

Goals	How to measure this goal	Scale
Fitness and co-ordination	Stamina (aerobic fitness)	low ➜ high level of stamina
	Strength	low ➜ high level of strength
	Flexibility (For these strategies, a group leader could use either informal observations or more formal measures of fitness such as BMI (body-mass index) test, blood pressure, heart rate measurement as appropriate)	low ➜ high level of flexibility
	Integration of body parts	poor ➜ good integration
	Contralateral patterning (i.e. arms swing in opposition to legs during walking)	poor ➜ good contralateral patterning
	Synchrony of body parts	arrhythmic ➜ rhythmic synchrony
The ability to relax	Release of muscle tension	high ➜ low muscular tension
	Release of psychological tension	agitated ➜ calm mental state
	Ability to transcend the moment through relaxation	inability ➜ ability to transcend
Connection between thought, imagination and body	Ability to explore a thought or feeling through expressive movement	unsuccessful ➜ successful movement exploration
Develop initiative, decision-making and leadership skills	Initiating activities	assisted ➜ independent initiation
	Making aesthetic decisions	assisted ➜ independent aesthetic decision-making
	Leading an activity	unsuccessful ➜ successful leadership
Performing skills	Focus in performance	Unfocused ➜ focused performance
	Ability to transform through performance	Inability ➜ ability to transform
	Confidence in performance	Unconfident ➜ confident performance
	Pleasure in performing	No pleasure ➜ pleasure

Table 10.3 could be used to assess the impact of a movement and dance program over time, for example, after participation for ten weeks or six months. Data required includes observations of movement based on the LMA framework, as well as formal and informal feedback from participants, families, carers and other professionals. Strategies for obtaining the latter kind of data are discussed below.

This table includes aspects of assessment and evaluation. Feder and Feder (1998) comment that these terms are often used interchangeably. In this context, however, we define assessment as relating to an individual's achievement. That is, how well a participant succeeded at what the program demanded of them. Evaluation, on the other hand, is more about what the program delivered. Did the program offer what that person wanted from it? What was their involvement like for them? Did they enjoy it? Did they feel that they learned something? We have included both aspects as it is equally important to discover how well an individual achieved what was desired, as it is to ascertain how successful a program is in delivering what was promised.

Strategies for obtaining verbal feedback

In addition to obtaining data through observation of movement, verbal feedback from stakeholders such as participants, parents/carers, other professionals can provide valuable insights. The following section details some strategies for obtaining feedback.

Informal feedback from participants

Participants can be offered informal opportunities to comment on their experience of participating in the group. These comments could be elicited by creating special times in class, perhaps in the last section before the formal goodbye. Questions like this could be used:

◉   What was the best thing we did today?

◉   Is there anything you didn't like about today's class?

◉   What would you like to do next time?

◉   Is there anything we haven't done that you would like to do?

This kind of questioning can be an effective strategy for those who have language and the confidence to express their thoughts and feelings. For those without language, it may be possible to elicit a non-verbal response. Some participants may prefer to use movement to express their feelings, as exemplified by this story about BreakOut member Erica. In this case, Jenny added her own verbal response to Erica's movement feedback to ensure that Erica's ability to communicate her feelings through movement was recognised.

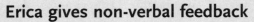

Erica gives non-verbal feedback

After a group improvisation based on the theme of a river, participants regrouped to discuss their experience. I (Jenny) facilitated the discussion by asking them what it felt like to 'be in the river'. Some members described their experience in words, saying 'it felt soft', 'It reminded me of the birds on the Yarra River', 'I liked it when it was fast', 'peaceful', 'bridges'.

When it was Erica's turn to describe her experience, she chose not to use words, even though she has competent language skills. Instead, she raised her arms above her head and reached to the ceiling. Then in slow motion her hands began to sway until the motion rippled through her arms and body. This took close to a minute to complete. Erica finished with a smile and said in a soft voice, 'river'. I acknowledged Erica's movement description by telling her about the feeling it gave me while I was watching her. 'Erica, watching you do that movement made me feel so peaceful. I was captivated by the way your body moved so slowly and freely. It reminded me of looking at the water on a calm day'. Again I asked Erica how it made her feel. Erica replied, 'Nice'.

Informal feedback from parents/carers

The process of understanding a participant's experience in the dance program can be helped by informal conversations with carers or families. A friendly question to a carer or parent who accompanies an individual to the program, such as, 'How do you think Neil is enjoying dance class?', may elicit valuable information about the person's response to the program as indicated in other areas of their life. For example, a family may hear comments about the program between sessions, or may observe that their child/client is keen to get up and moving on the day of the program. These observations may not necessarily be positive. For example, a carer may notice that a participant seems to become overtired after attending a program in hot weather.

Formal questionnaires

It can be useful to provide participants and families/carers with the opportunity to offer their opinions about the program and its impact in a more formal way, such as a questionnaire offered periodically, perhaps at the end of a term or year. This allows for a more considered response and the possibility of anonymous comments, which can be more comfortable for both parties, especially if the feedback is critical. A questionnaire can assist in obtaining feedback about participants' and families'/carers' responses to content of the program, as well as that about management and administrative issues. The questionnaire should be brief and easy to answer for those with limited time or interest (multiple choice options are best for this purpose). It should also include space for additional comments. A sample questionnaire used at BreakOut appears as Appendix B. Feedback opportunities should also be made available to other stakeholders, including other staff, professionals and program hosts.

A tool for assessing an individual's response to a dance program

The tool that appears as Appendix C has been developed as a means of assessing an individual's response and progress as a result of participation in a dance program. It is not about comparison between people or measurement against any external standard. What might be an apathetic response for a motivated participant, may be a level of involvement higher than that shown for other activities for participant who has difficulty engaging. A group leader would hope to see development of individual participants in a range of areas including expansion of movement capabilities, enjoyment, creative expression and a sense of connection to the group. All of these are only relevant in comparison with the previous state of that particular individual. In order to assess an individual's response, the group leader needs to:

- Decide on goals to be evaluated. These should be commensurate with both the stated goals of the program and those of participants.
- Plan a session that will include opportunities for progress towards each of these goals to be demonstrated. For example, if leadership skills are to be evaluated, then the session must include activities in which participants can demonstrate leadership.
- Offer participants, parents, carers and other stakeholders the opportunity to respond to a questionnaire about their perception of the program.
- Create an evaluation chart (as per Appendix C) for each participant that includes all relevant goals and measures.
- Run the session, ideally with at least one evaluator who is not involved in leading activities.
- If there is more than one evaluator, then compare notes and discuss differences in observations
- Create a report based on a consensus of observers, as well as information gained from questionnaires of participants and other stakeholders.
- Discuss the final report with relevant parties. Consider any changes that need to be made to improve participants' achievement and enjoyment of the program.
- Celebrate the success and achievement of participants and the program.

Self-monitoring and evaluation: Reflective practice

As well as monitoring participants' progress and the responses of all stakeholders to the program, it is important for a professional to continually monitor and develop their skills and techniques. Some strategies that a group leader might employ for this include:

- keeping a journal of the program, including a record of activities that worked and areas for improvement
- holding discussion and feedback sessions with other staff members
- video-recording sessions as a means of monitoring one's own actions, particularly those movement patterns and behaviours that may be unconscious

◉ arranging a program of professional supervision, 'an opportunity to discuss and receive feedback on therapeutic work for the purpose of professional growth and accountability' (Murrow, 1998). Supervision possibilities are varied and may include informal or formal conversations with supervisors or colleagues, the use of videotaped sessions, role play, facilitated movement exploration of specific themes and issues for therapists in their development (Murrow, 1998). Dance therapy and some dance education training include at least some supervision as part of the core program.

◉ regularly attending professional development activities: conferences, workshops, training sessions, to learn new skills and refresh old ones.

A class member inadvertently gives feedback on an unconscious habit

I (Jenny) became aware of my frequent use of 'OK?' at the end of sentences when a young class member with autism began to use this pattern of speech as he verbally anticipated my introduction of each new activity. This was quite an amusing way to receive feedback about my unconscious habit!

Response: After evaluation, then what?

There must be development or change if the process of evaluation of a program is to have any value. The group leader's actions in response to information obtained through evaluation could be:

◉ to consider participants' progress as assessed and adjust the program accordingly, adding activities to improve areas of participants' weakness, reducing or modifying activities that are not enjoyed and expanding on those that are.

◉ To reconsider participants' and other stakeholders' stated motivations for involvement in the program to ensure that these are being met.

Dissemination of findings

The final stage of evaluation is the dissemination of results to all stakeholders and other relevant parties. Relevant information could be sent to funding bodies which may be interested in funding the project in the future. A summary of comments received from participants, families and carers could appear in the group's newsletter, as well as the program leader's response and plans for change. Program host organisations may be interested in measured outcomes as well as participants' self-reports of enjoyment and learning through the program.

Challenges of evaluation

Having described a range of strategies for the process of evaluation, we must acknowledge the considerable challenges dance group leaders are likely to face when they consider undertaking evaluation. For many people working as sessional leaders, either as therapists, teachers or community artists, there may be little opportunity for paid time to undertake any kind of evaluative process. There may also be little interest from the host organisation in the goals or measurement of outcomes of the dance program. This seems to be particularly so in the case of the disability sector in Australia. The culture of other settings such as hospitals, early intervention centres and rehabilitation programs are much more focused on the evaluation of outcomes.

There is also the problem that too much focus on evaluation can detract from the main purpose of a dance program, which may be the provision of an enjoyable and expressive experience. With some groups, particularly those with high support needs, there are often not large changes or breakthroughs even with constant quality input. A big focus on achievement in a dance program might serve to emphasise group members' disabilities and lead to a feeling of disillusionment among hardworking and committed staff.

This is not to say that evaluation should not occur, but a group leader may keep these issues in mind when considering what, if any, process of evaluation should take place.

Conclusion

Freedom to Move is our contribution to the legitimation of the value of movement and dance for people with intellectual disabilities. We hope it will serve to:

◉ increase interest in participation in dance programs from people with intellectual disabilities, their parents and carers

◉ motivate more skilled dance group leaders to become interested in the disability field

◉ help those leaders do a better job, faster and for longer (i.e. save them from having to learn everything from their own experience so they don't burn-out so quickly)

◉ help those leaders become more effective advocates for their profession

◉ inspire more policy-makers and managers to be convinced of the value of movement and dance for their organisations and to direct more resources to it.

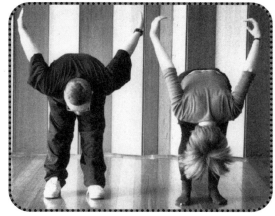

We urge other practitioners and therapists to take action; do further study, undertake research to add to the evidence base for this field, present at conferences, publish articles and books! And most of all, enjoy dancing!

Glossary

articulation: In reference to movement, articulation means awareness of and the capacity to move areas of the body separately. For example, articulating the spine would mean feeling or moving each vertebra in the spine separately.

attunement: A technique used by dance therapists to identify with an individual and offer comfort and affirmation of an individual's experience of themselves through movement. It is the process of the therapist responsively duplicating changes in muscle tension of a mover (Loman and Merman, 1996), and can be considered similar to kinaesthetic empathy. Attunement relies on intuition and is a means of communicating that needs no words. Using attunement to share another person's experience is about creating a safe, permissive and non-judgmental environment. A dance therapist would use attunement to 'start where that person is' and establish a deep empathic rapport. This concept is really the opposite of the behaviour modification approach that is so much part of the life experience of many people with disabilities. Being attuned to another person is more about getting into their shoes than getting them to change their shoes.

attuned energy: Related to attunement. When the movement relationship of a duo or group is complementary and harmonious. It may not necessarily be exactly the same, but sufficiently alike or attuned that the movers feel comfortable together.

autism: A developmental disability. A person with autism will have significant difficulties in several areas of their development. The areas most affected are communication, social interaction and behaviour. This developmental disability may have a particular pattern called autism, or there may be varying amounts of disability in other areas of development which result in patterns called Asperger syndrome or Pervasive Developmental Disorder – Not Otherwise Specified (PDD – NOS). This whole area of developmental disabilities is referred to as Autism Spectrum Disorders. People with these disorders are affected differently, but all require specialised assistance and support. See also www.autismaus.com.au (Australia), www.autism.co.uk (UK), www.autism-society.org (USA).

canon: A technique in which one dancer's movement is repeated exactly by a series of other dancers in quick succession, roughly equivalent to a Mexican Wave.

clashing energy: When the energy connection between partners or group of movers clashes and is inharmonious.

co-active assistance: Hands-on facilitation of movement by a staff member in consultation with the participant. Some people, especially those who are less mobile because of a physical disability, may need this kind of involvement from a staff member. This allows for a fuller engagement in activities and can make movement easier. A relationship of trust between the participant and the staff member is required if the experience is to be non-intrusive for the participant.

community arts: A model of art-making that 'celebrates the diversity and talents of people in the community … whose value is to build and express diverse community cultures, as part of the culture of wider society' (Williams, 2001).

Constructive Rest Pose (CRP): The safest position for lying on the floor, one that reduces pressure on the spine and neck, and allows the spine to flatten out comfortably. The person lies with their back flat on the floor, knees together, bent up at a 90-degree angle and feet placed flat on the floor about 60 cm apart. Hands and arms are flat on the floor, palms face up, or down as desired.

Creative dance: 'A free approach to the art of body movement which gives everyone opportunity to discover for himself his own forms of movement expression according to his physiological and psychological needs' (Mettler, 1990, p. 95).

dance therapy (often used interchangeably with term **dance/movement therapy**): '[T]he psychotherapeutic use of movement as a process which furthers the emotional, cognitive, social and physical integration of the individual. Dance/Movement therapists work with individuals who have social, emotional, cognitive and/or physical problems. They are employed in psychiatric hospitals, clinics, day care, community mental health centers, developmental centers, correctional facilities, special schools and rehabilitation facilities. They work with people of all ages in both groups and individually. They act as consultants and engage in research' (www.adta.org)

developmental movement patterns: These are 'based on the natural development and unfolding of potential within the human being' (Hartley, 1995) and were developed by American dancer, occupational therapist and movement educator Bonnie Bainbridge Cohen, as part of the movement theory known as Body–Mind Centering. These principles acknowledge that:

◎ there are differences in the timing and progress of each child's physical skills and co-ordination, and that this needs to be taken into account when planning a dance program.

◎ human movement development occurs in a layered fashion. Early movement patterns such as sitting, rolling, creeping, crawling, etc. underlie and support the emergence of more sophisticated movement patterns such as walking, running, jumping, skipping, turning. To assist children to master more complex movement skills, we return to earlier movement patterns to support their development (adapted from Wishart 2000).

Down syndrome: A genetic condition caused by extra material on chromosome 21, one of the most frequent causes of intellectual disability. People with Down syndrome can have a broad range of ability from profoundly disabled to low/average intelligence, however, most children with Down syndrome have mild to moderate learning difficulties. The person who has Down syndrome has far more normal characteristics than abnormal characteristics. They also inherit genes from both sides of the family and so have family characteristics and family resemblances. Some common traits include low muscle tone, legs and arms shorter in relation to the torso, a cleft between the first and second toes and delays in reaching milestones, e.g. sitting, crawling, talking, toileting, etc. See also www.dsav.asn.au (Australia), www.nads.org (USA), www.downs-syndrome.org.uk (UK).

echolalia: Characteristic behaviour of some people with autism; automatic repetition of words and phrases, particularly those just heard, but may include stored information (Miller, 1984).

Effort: the aspect of Laban framework of movement that describes how movement occurs, the amount of energy used and how it is released. Effort is comprised of four elements: Flow, Weight, Space and Time.

hypotonic: low muscle tone, as indicated by floppy or weak musculature, common in people with Down syndrome.

improvisation: The art of improvisation as it is practised in the twenty-first century developed out of modern dance. Improvisation is about opening up to impulse and tapping into the subconscious without intellectual censorship. It allows spontaneous and simultaneous exploring, creating and performing (Blom and Chaplin 1988, p. ix). Nachmanovitch (1990, p. 9) describes it as 'the master key to creativity'. In improvised dance, participants and audiences appreciate the shapes and movements created spontaneously in response to the energy and mood present in the group.

in the moment: To be fully present and aware of what is happening right now, in that particular moment. This concept is particularly important in improvised artforms which require participants to be fully present to the immediate situation and capable of reacting to the unexpected.

independent: In this context, independent means individuals who are capable of initiating movement, who have cognitive skills to process basic information and who are able to work co-operatively in a group.

intellectual disability: To be considered intellectually disabled, an individual must have an IQ of below 70, and have everyday life skills, including personal skills such as self-care and communication, that are inadequate when compared with others of the same age and culture. These two conditions must be present prior to the age of 18 years. It is estimated that approximately one per cent of the Australian population has an intellectual disability. About three-quarters of these are in the mild range, while the rest are moderate, severe or profound. The majority of cases have no identifiable reason, although Down syndrome is the most frequently identifiable cause (DHS, 1997).

Laban: Rudolf Laban (1879–1958) was a pioneer in movement education and modern dance, who has had a very significant impact on the development of dance practice in the early to mid-twentieth century, initially in Europe and the United Kingdom. Later his thinking and writing influenced dance around the world, as the value of his framework in dance-related fields, such as education, therapy, notation, research and choreography, became manifest. Laban's work continues to this day at the Laban Centre in London, through training in dance, dance therapy and related disciplines, and by numerous other institutions and practitioners whose activities have been informed by a new way of looking at dance and movement.

layering: A technique used in improvisational dance in which a dance or choreography is created by a gradual adding of layers of complexity

LMA (Laban Movement Analysis) 'A language based on a way of seeing the world which describes all human movement, whether it be movement behaviour, the way the body functions or how we express ourselves' (Leah, 2000). This system is useful for the quantitative and qualitative measurement of human movement. The basic concepts on which this movement language are based are outlined briefly in Chapter 2, i.e. Body, Space, Effort (comprised of Time, Weight, Flow and Space) and Relationship. Laban's original concepts have been expanded by others, most notably by Irmgard Bartenieff, who developed the overarching conceptual framework for analysing and synthesising human movement studies that has become known as LMA. For more about LMA, see Moore and Yamamoto (1988) and Dell (1977).

mirroring: A therapeutic method of establishing and maintaining a relationship that involves the therapist's accurate observation and execution of the client's movement behaviour so as to convey understanding and acceptance; unlike 'copying', mirroring may reflect only the salient elements of the movement, thereby working to focus on treatment goals (Freundlich, Pike and Schwartz, 1989, p. 51).

normalisation: Principles for people with learning disabilities that include the right to the same opportunities in the community as others; greater independence as part of an age appropriate lifestyle; involvement in decisions affecting their own lives; and provision of services that are local, accessible and comprehensive (Carnaby, 1999).

Relationship: one of the four concepts of the Laban movement framework on which the dance practice in this book is based. Relationship is about the connection with other people and/or objects through movement. This can be a relationship between body parts, different movements and shapes, individuals and groups, as well as the environment. Some concepts it encompasses include towards and away from, around, through, between, over and under, before and after, faster and slower, alike and different.

social capital: The institutions, relationships, and norms that shape the quality and quantity of a society's social interactions. Increasing evidence shows that social cohesion is critical for societies to prosper economically and for development to be sustainable. Social capital is not just the sum of the institutions which underpin a society – it is the glue that holds them together (www.worldbank.org).

special needs: In discussing children with special needs, we mean children whose development is in some way impaired or delayed, and who need more than regular education and care. This term is now being replaced by 'additional needs', indicating that children are not qualitatively different from others, but that they have some needs that are additional to those of most children. These children may or may not have intellectual disabilities as adults.

transform: To be changed in form or substance (*Chambers Dictionary*). In this context transform/transformation means, that through dance, an individual's experience of themselves, or another's perception of them is in some way changed.

Appendix A

The BreakOut Dance Group Story

www.breakoutdancegroup.com

BreakOut is a community-based dance group that provides weekly creative dance classes specifically for people with intellectual disabilities. BreakOut also provides social and performing opportunities in community activities, such as festivals and special events, and special projects in other areas of the arts, such as film-making projects with artists in residence.

BreakOut caters for children, teenagers and adults in three separate age-specific groups. The weekly sessions are led by one of the directors, both qualified dance teacher/therapists, supported by a professionally trained assistant, and community and student volunteers. BreakOut is based in Moorabbin, a southern suburb of Melbourne, Australia.

BreakOut began in 1991 under the umbrella of Cadance Community Dance Group in Malvern. The group was founded and directed by Marita Smith until 1996. Karen Ermacora led the group in 1997, and Kim Dunphy and Jenny Scott have shared the leadership role since 1997.

BreakOut's aims are three-fold:

1   Improved health and wellbeing for individual participants by encouraging the development of:

- physical fitness and body awareness
- social connectedness
- creative self-expression and spontaneity
- self-esteem
- independent and group work skills e.g. co-operation, negotiation, contribution and decision-making

2   Development and dissemination of specialist knowledge and skills in the field of dance for people with disabilities.

BreakOut provides education and training in the area of dance and disability through:

- student placements (special education, physiotherapy, dance therapy, creative arts therapy and disability studies students)
- professional development workshops
- conference presentations
- journal publications.

3   Community awareness

BreakOut aims to raise community awareness of the creative potential of people with intellectual disabilities through:

- performance in mainstream and specialised events and festivals
- involvement in professional organisations such as Ausdance Victoria Community Dance Working Group and the Dance Therapy Association of Australia.

BreakOut aims to contribute to community awareness of the value of the arts as a tool for development of wellbeing through:

- advocacy with government, disability and community agencies
- professional development for workers in the field as in (2) above
- publication as in (2) above.

Appendix B

BreakOut Dance Group Inc.

Member survey   Date

We would be pleased if you could tell us what you like about BreakOut and anything we might improve on.

NAME: (Optional, be anonymous if you like) _

These questions are about the content of our program. Please think about the things you/your child/client does in class when answering them. Circle the number that best approximates your opinion.

How important are these aspects of BreakOut for you?

Fun: enjoying myself

1. Not at all   2. Not much   3. A little   4. Somewhat   5. A lot

Fitness: keeping fit

1. Not at all   2. Not much   3. A little   4. Somewhat   5. A lot

Friendship: making new friends or enjoying the company of old friends

1. Not at all   2. Not much   3. A little   4. Somewhat   5. A lot

Creativity: having the chance to express myself

1. Not at all   2. Not much   3. A little   4. Somewhat   5. A lot

Other? (please describe)

_____

1. Not at all   2. Not much   3. A little   4. Somewhat   5. A lot

How well do you think BreakOut classes fulfil those needs?

Fun: I enjoy myself at BreakOut

1. Not at all   2. Not much   3. A little   4. Somewhat   5. A lot

Fitness: BreakOut helps me keep fit

1. Not at all   2. Not much   3. A little   4. Somewhat   5. A lot

Friendship: BreakOut gives me a chance to make new friends and catch up with old friends

1. Not at all   2. Not much   3. A little   4. Somewhat   5. A lot

Creativity: BreakOut gives me the chance to express myself

1. Not at all   2. Not much   3. A little   4. Somewhat   5. A lot

Other?: (please describe)

_____

1. Not at all   2. Not much   3. A little   4. Somewhat   5. A lot

Comments

_____
_____
_____
_____

For you, what are the best things about coming to Break Out?

_____
_____
_____
_____
_____

What are the worst things about coming to BreakOut?

_____

_____

_____

_____

_____

Is there anything you think we should do better or differently?

_____

_____

_____

_____

Any other comments?

_____

_____

_____

_____

PROGRAM MANAGEMENT

The following questions are about the management of our program.

VENUE

Do you find this venue easily accessible?

1. Not at all   2. Not much   3. A little   4. Somewhat   5. A lot

Do you think this venue is suitable and safe for BreakOut class members?

1. Not at all   2. Not much   3. A little   4. Somewhat   5. A lot

TIME-TABLING

Does the current timetabling of classes suit you?

1. Not at all   2. Not much   3. A little   4. Somewhat   5. A lot

If not, when would you prefer classes to be held?

_____

_____

_____

COST

Do you find the program value for money?

1. Not at all   2. Not much   3. A little   4. Somewhat   5. A lot

Is it difficult for you to find the money for the program?

1. Not at all   2. Not much   3. A little   4. Somewhat   5. A lot

Any other comments?

_____

_____

_____

_____

Thank you for your time. We appreciate receiving your comments and will consider them to help us keep doing our best at BreakOut.

Jenny Scott,
Co-ordinator

Appendix C

Sample tool for evaluation of an individual's participation in a dance program

Date		Participant's name:
		Evaluator's name:
Goal to be evaluated	**How to measure it**	**Scale**
A sense of fun and enjoyment	Informal reports from parents and carers	Antipathy ➔ enjoyment 1. antipathy 2. not much enjoyment 3. a little 4. some 5. great enjoyment
	Informal feedback in class	Antipathy ➔ enjoyment 1. antipathy 2. not much enjoyment 3. a little 4. some 5. great enjoyment
	Surveys	Antipathy ➔ enjoyment 1. antipathy 2. not much enjoyment 3. a little 4. some 5. great enjoyment
	Observation of non-verbal behaviour; (facial expression, body stance, relationship)	Displeasure ➔ smiling 1. no smiling 2. not much 3. a little 4. some 5. a lot of smiling Body tension ➔ ease 1. a lot of tension 2. some tension 3. neutral tension 4. some ease 5. great ease Distress (withdrawal, crying, emotional outburst, physical agitation e.g. flapping, rocking, masturbation, dangerous or self-harming behaviour) ➔ playfulness 1. very distressed 2. a little distressed 3. no distress 4. quite playful 5. very playful
	Observation of verbal/ vocalisations	Verbally non -communicative (silent, withdrawn) ➔ communicative (laughing , talking, spontaneous comments) 1. non-communicative 2. not very communicative 3. a little 4. quite 5. very communicative
	Attendance record	Infrequent ➔ regular attendance 1. infrequent attendance 2. sporadic 3. fairly regular 4. regular 5. very regular attendance

	Level of involvement	Low ➜ high level of involvement 1. very uninvolved 2. quite uninvolved 3. neutral 4. quite involved 5. very involved
	Level of enthusiasm	Apathy ➜ high level of enthusiasm 1. very apathetic 2. a little apathetic 3. neutral 4. quite enthusiastic 5. very enthusiastic
Connection with the here and now	Focus on group activity	distracted (physically restless, scattered attention, inward focus) ➜ focused energy 1. very distracted energy 2. partly distracted energy 3. neutral 4. partly focused 5. very focused energy
	Energy attuned appropriately to the activity	clashing ➜ attuned energy 1. very clashing energy 2. some clashing 3. neutral 4. some attunement 5. very attuned energy
Connection and communication with others	Non-verbal communication energy attuned appropriately to partner or group	Clashing ➜ attuned energy 1. very clashing energy 2. some clashing 3. neutral 4. some attunement 5. very attuned energy
	Eye contact	Inappropriate ➜ appropriate 1. very inappropriate 2. quite inappropriate 3. neutral 4. quite appropriate 5. very appropriate
	Use of personal space	Inappropriate ➜ appropriate 1. very inappropriate 2. quite inappropriate 3. neutral 4. quite appropriate 5. very appropriate
	Initiation of contact	Unsuccessful ➜ successful 1. very unsuccessful 2. quite unsuccessful 3. neutral 4. quite successful 5. very successful
	Sustainment of contact	Unsuccessful ➜ successful 1. very unsuccessful 2. quite unsuccessful 3. neutral 4. quite successful 5. very successful
	Release of contact	Unsuccessful ➜ successful 1. very unsuccessful 2. quite unsuccessful 3. neutral 4. quite successful 5. very successful
	Turn-taking	Unsuccessful ➜ successful 1. very unsuccessful 2. quite unsuccessful 3. neutral 4. quite successful 5. very successful
	Physical contact	Inappropriate ➜ appropriate 1. very inappropriate 2. quite inappropriate 3. neutral 4. quite appropriate 5. very appropriate

	Verbal communication expressive verbal interaction	Inexpressive ➜ expressive 1. very inexpressive 2. quite inexpressive 3. neutral 4. quite expressive 5. very expressive
	Appropriate verbal interaction: listening, turn-taking, empathising	Inappropriate ➜ appropriate 1. very inappropriate 2. quite inappropriate 3. neutral 4. quite appropriate 5. very appropriate
	Confidence in self-expression (verbal and non-verbal)	Unconfident ➜ confident expression of personal feelings and experiences 1. very unconfident 2. quite unconfident 3. neutral 4. quite confident 5. very confident
Body awareness, mastery and expansion of movement range	Articulation of body parts Upper: (head, shoulders, arms, hands)	Low ➜ high level of articulation 1. very poor articulation 2. poor articulation 3. neutral 4. some articulation 5. very good articulation
	Centre: (abdominals, chest, pelvis, spine)	Low ➜ high level of articulation 1. very poor articulation 2. poor articulation 3. neutral 4. some articulation 5. very good articulation
	Lower: (legs, knees, ankles, feet)	Low ➜ high level of articulation 1. very poor articulation 2. poor articulation 3. neutral 4. some articulation 5. very good articulation
	Extremities: (arms, wrist, fingers)	Low ➜ high level of articulation 1. very poor articulation 2. poor articulation 3. neutral 4. some articulation 5. very good articulation
	Use of space: (near, mid, reach, far)	Restricted➜ expansive 1. very restricted 2. restrictedn 3. neutral 4. expansive 5. very expansive
	Access to effort qualities: flow (bound-free)	Low ➜ high level of access to range of flow qualities 1. very poor access 2. poor access 3. neutral 4. reasonable access 5. very good access

	Space (direct – indirect)	Low ➜ high level of access to range of dimensions in space 1. very poor access 2. poor access 3. neutral 4. reasonable access 5. very good access
	Weight (light – strong)	Low ➜ high level of access to weight variations 1. very poor access 2. poor access 3. neutral 4. reasonable access 5. very good access
	Time (sustained – sudden)	Low ➜ high level of access to time variations 1. very poor access 2. poor access 3. neutral 4. reasonable access 5. very good access
Fitness and co-ordination	Stamina (aerobic fitness)	Low ➜ high level of stamina 1. very poor stamina 2. poor stamina 3. neutral 4. reasonable stamina 5. very good stamina
	Strength	low ➜ high level of strength 1. very weak 2. quite weak 3. neutral 4. quite strong 5. very strong
	Flexibility (For these strategies, a group leader could use either informal observations or more formal measures of fitness such as BMI (body-mass index) test, blood pressure, heart rate measurement) as appropriate.	Low ➜ high level of flexibility 1. very unflexible 2. quite unflexible 3. neutral 4. quite flexible 5. very flexible
	Integration of body parts	Poor ➜ good integration 1. very poor integration 2. poor integration 3. neutral 4. reasonable integration 5. very good integration
	Contralateral patterning (i.e. arms swing in opposition to legs during walking)	Poor ➜ good contralateral patterning 1. very poor patterning 2. poor patterning 3. neutral 4. reasonable 5. very good
	Rhythmic synchrony of body parts (body parts move with traditional integration and flow)	Arrhythmic ➜ rhythmic synchrony 1. very arrhythmic 2. quite arrhythmic 3. neutral 4. reasonably rhythmic 5. very rhythmic

The ability to relax	Release of muscle tension	High ➔ low muscle tension 1. very tense 2. quite tense 3. neutral 4. quite relaxed 5. very relaxed
	Release of psychological tension	Agitated ➔ calm mental state 1. very agitated 2. quite agitated 3. neutral 4. reasonably calm 5. very calm
	Ability to transcend the moment through relaxation	Inability ➔ ability to transcend 1. no ability to transcend 2. little ability 3. neutral 4. some ability 5. very able to transcend
Connection between thought, imagination and body	Ability to explore a thought or feeling through expressive movement	Inability ➔ ability to explore through movement 1. no ability 2. little ability 3. neutral 4. some ability 5. very able Unsuccessful ➔ successful movement exploration 1. very unsuccessful 2. quite unsuccessful 3. neutral 4. quite successful 5. very successful
Develop initiative, decision making and leadership skills	Initiating activities	Assisted ➔ independent initiation 1. needs much assistance 2. needs a little assistance 3. neutral 4. quite independent 5. very independent
	Make aesthetic decisions	Assisted ➔ independent aesthetic decision making 1. needs much assistance 2. needs a little assistance 3. neutral 4. quite independent 5. very independent
	Leading an activity	Unsuccessful ➔ successful leadership 1. very unsuccessful 2. quite unsuccessful 3. neutral 4. successful 5. very successful
Performing skills	Focus in performance	Unfocused ➔ focused performance 1. very unfocused 2. quite unfocused 3. neutral 4. quite focused 5. very focused
	Ability to transform through performance	Inability ➔ ability to transform 1. no ability to transform 2. little ability 3. neutral 4. some ability 5. very able to transform
	Confidence in performance	Unconfident ➔ confident performance 1. very unconfident 2. underconfident 3. neutral 4. reasonably confident 5. very confident
	Pleasure in performing	No pleasure ➔ pleasure 1. no pleasure 2. not much pleasure 3. neutral 4. some pleasure 5. much pleasure

Appendix D

Organisations: Dance, therapy and disability arts organisations

Dance

Ausdance (Australian Dance Council)

Ausdance is the national peak body for dance in Australia, with branches in each state and territory. Many branches have a sub-committee or interest group focused on dance in the community. The Victorian branch for example, has a community dance interest group.

dance.com.unity

www.ausdance.org.au

National Dance Association, USA

The mission of the National Dance Association is to increase knowledge, improve skills, and encourage sound professional practices in dance education while promoting and supporting creative and healthy lifestyles through high quality dance programs.

www.aahperd.org/nda

Foundation for Community Dance, UK

The industry's lead body for community dance, working for the development of dance for all.

www.communitydance.org.uk

www.danceuk.org

Disability arts

e-bility.com - Arts, Worldwide

Resources for people with disabilities who are interested in art and creative programs such as dance, painting, drama and music.

www.e-bility.com/links/arts.htm

DADAA (Disability in the Arts, Disadvantage in the Arts Australia)

The peak body for arts and disability, arts and disadvantage in Australia.

www.dadaanat.net.au

Arts Access

This is the Victorian branch of a DADAA, providing training, information, networking, database, support, library publications

www.artsaccess.com.au/

Very Special Arts, USA

International organisation providing opportunities for people with disabilities to express themselves and learn by getting involved in the arts www.vsarts.org

National Disability Arts Forum, UK

Aims to promote the participation of disabled persons in art.

www.ndaf.org

London Disability Arts Forum, UK

Organisation that aims to promote the arts among disabled people.

www.dail.dircon.co.uk

Northern Disability Arts Forum, UK

Self-managed service promoting the arts for disabled people in Tyne and Wear, Cleveland, Cumbria, Durham, and Northumberland.

www.stare.net/nordaf/index.htm

Dance therapy

International Institute for Dance Therapy, Worldwide

www.dancetherapy.com

Dance Therapy Association of Australia
Peak body for dance therapy in Australia www.dtaa.org

Association for Dance Movement Therapy, UK www.dmtuk.demon.co.uk

American Dance Therapy Association, USA www.adta.org

Brecha -Dance Movement Therapy en Argentina www.brecha.com.ar

German Dance Therapy Association www.dancetherapy.de

Japan Dance Therapy Association www.asahi-net.or.jp

Netherlands: Hogeschool voor muziek en dans www.hmd.nl

Spanish Dance Movement Therapy Association (ADMTE)
www.danzamovimientoterapia.com:

Arts in Therapy Network www.artsintherapy.com

Expressive Therapy Concepts www.expressivetherapy.org

Voice of Dance www.voiceofdance.com

Resources

Arts in Psychotherapy Journal at www/elsevier.nl/locate/issn/01974556

At Health Newsletter at www.athealth.com

Dye-namic Movement Products www.dyenamicmovement.com

IDEA (Institute for the Development of Educational Activities, Inc.) www.IDEA.org

Folk dance resources

Folk Dance Australia

Folk dance resources including videos, music and instruction booklets are available from Folk Dance Australia, www.geocities.com/Vienna/4677

AVDP World Dance

AVDP World Dance offers a range of folk dance resources including videos, recorded music and dance instructions. Ph: Australia (61) 02 9528 4813 or Okaye@optusnet.com.au

Shenanigans

Shenanigans is a folk dance band that sells a range of CDs with instruction books of dance suitable for adults and children's groups. 'The Phoenix Special', for example, includes Macedonian, German, Yiddish, Romanian, French, Hungarian, Indonesian and Greek dances to assist the teaching of music, dance and social concepts. Ph: 03 9406 7980, email: shenanigan@optusnet.com.au or www.shenanigansmusic.com.au

Victorian Orff Schulwerk Association

The Victorian Orff Schulwerk Association sells a range of excellent resources, runs professional development workshops especially relevant for people interested in the connection between music and dance. www.VOSA.org.au

Folk Dance Association

Folk Dance Association provides services and information for folk dancers, folk dance leaders and folk dance groups throughout the United States and Canada.

www.folkdancing.org

Appendix E

Discography

World music

Saltwater Band, *Gapu Damurrun*, www.skinnyfishmusic.com.au (1998)
Lively rhythmic tracks by Australian aboriginal band

Various artists, *World Playground,* Putumayo Music (2000)
Angelique Kidjo, *Ayé*, Island Records, Phonogram (1994)
Lively African pop-rock

Tribal Trance, Minjarah (1998)
Excellent selection from flowing to strong rhythms

Various artists, *Afro Latino*, Putumayo Music (1998)
Rhythmic and joyful African and Latin music

Mickey Hart, *Planet Drum,* Rykodisc (1991)
Great drumming music and vocals

Martin Cradick, Su Hart and Baka Forest People from Congo, *Spirit of the Forest: Baka Beyond*, Festival Music (1995)
lively African tracks for warm-up and vigorous dancing

Café del Mar, *Arias 2: New Horizon*, Ibiza, Reach Music
Mellow And subdued

Thula Sana, *Thula Sana*, self produced, Melbourne
Medium tempo lively African tunes

Gypsy Soul, *New Flamenco*, Narada Productions (1999)
Flowing rhythms; great to get the arms and legs moving

Theo Dorakis, *Zorba's Dance*, lcd EMI
Modern disco style Greek music for circle and travelling dances

Mikis Theodorakis, *Zorba the Greek* (soundtrack)
Very lively music for Greek style circle and travelling dances

'Morrison's Jig' and 'The Brown Jug Polka', Shenanigans, *International Bush Dancing,*
Shenanigans
Bush dance music

Various artists, *A Jewish Odyssey*, Putumayo World Music
'Dancing on Water', 'Meron Nigun', *Klezmania,* Oystralia, www.klezmania.com.au
Lively Israeli and Klezmer style music

Bando Tropicana E Benedito Costa, *Lambada: Latin Disco*,
Blackboard: West Germany (1987)
Lively Latin music; good for getting big groups moving in a line

Hot Toddy, *Celtic Fire*, Hart Records (1999)
Riverdance soundtrack
Fast moving Irish music

Disco & Pop

Abba, *Abba Gold: Greatest Hits*, Polar Music (1992)
Simple rhythm, favourite songs to sing-along

'Blue Suede Shoes', 'Hound Dog", *Elvis, Disco De Ouro*, Summit
Elvis' most famous disco-style songs

Various artists, *The Best Ever Disco Album*, EMI Music Australia (1998)
Extensive range of disco songs on double CD

'Love Is In the Air', 'Perhaps, Perhaps', 'Time After Time', John Paul Young and other
artists, *Strictly Ballroom* soundtrack
A great CD for dancing which includes music for ballroom, disco and Spanish dance

'Kokomo', 'Don't Worry, Be Happy', Various artists, *Cocktail* soundtrack,
WEA: Elektra Entertainment (1988)
Easy paced sing-along songs

Rock'n'roll style

'Good Golly Miss Molly', 'Be-Bop-A-Lula', Various artists, *Hooked On Rock'n'Roll*,
Music World: Hughes Leisure Group
'All Shook Up', *Elvis Presley*, Presley, RCA
Many old rock'n'roll favourites

The Commitments, *The Commitments* (soundtrack), MCA records
'Mustang Sally' is a great track to get everyone rocking!
Rock-style

Tracks 5, 7 and 9, 'Jambalaya', 'Tit Galop' and 'Pig Ankle Rag', *Jugularity Greatest Hats*,
Jugularity, www. jugularity.com (1996)
Lively travelling music suitable for gallops, runs,

Social dance music

Various artists, *The Bird Dance and other Party Favourites*, Master Sounds (1998)
Simple well-known social dances

Track 9, 'Honky Tonk Blues', Various artists, *Line Dance: The Ultimate Collection*,
Liberty Records:EMI (1994)
Country and western style dance music

Mellow ballads and country music

'Lucille', 'Singing My Song', Tammy Wynette, *Country Music Giants*,
Hughes Leisure Group
Shania Twain, Shania Twain
Well-known sing-along favourites

'Island Home', Christine Anu, *Stylin' Up*
Indigenous Australian rock singer

'Ode to My Family', The Cranberries, *No Need To Argue*, Island Records (1994)
Great to hum along to

'Do Right Woman', 'Natural Woman', Aretha Franklin, *Best of Aretha Franklin*
Songs with a with a nice sway

Billie Holliday, *Best of Billie Holliday*, Sony Music (1990)
Slow paced mellow blues

Familiar music/easy listening
Good for gentle movement and sing alongs

Elton John, *The Very Best of Elton John*, Happenstance Ltd (1990)
Tom Jones, *Greatest Hits of Tom Jones*, HiFi label (1992)
Recommended for lifting a mood on a sombre day

'Song Sung Blue', 'Sweet Caroline' 'Cracklin Rosie', 'Blue Jeans', *Neil Diamond The Ultimate Collection*, Columbia
Medium tempo favourite sing-along especially for older adults

'What A Wonderful World', Louis Armstrong, *What A Wonderful World*
Great album of old favourites, mostly lively, also good for singing along

Classical/mellow
For stretches/quieter warm-up activities

Alice Gomez, *Flute Dreams*, TalkingTaco Music Inc. (1994)
Compositions that reflect the cultural heritage of the native peoples of the Americas

'Fur Elise', Brahms Waltz in A Flat major, Various artists, *Best of Romantic Piano Music*, Naxos Collection 18: Classic for Kids (1994)

J.S. Bach, Solo and Double Violin Concertos, Harmonia Mundi: France (1997)

Track 5, Marisa Robles, *The World of the Harp*, Decca (1992)
Ambient harp music, ideal for a slowing down activity

Jan Garbeck & the Hilliard Ensemble, *Officium*, ECM Records (1994)

Café del Mar, *Arias 2*, New Horizon: Paul Schwartz (1999)
Gentle and haunting music

Improvisation

Steve Falk, *The Marimba Project,* sfalk@iprimus.com.au (2000)
Interesting free form marimba music, great for nature/environment/sea themes

Vann Tiersen, *Amelie* soundtrack, Claude Ossard & UGC (2001)
Floating and mellow

'China on a Bicycle', *Southern Crossings*, Southern Crossings
Is a favourite track- lovely for mirroring activities and slow stretches

Jean-Michel Jarre, *Oxygene* (1993)
David Bowie, *A Space Odyssey* (2001)
Ambient, other worldly

Cirque du Soleil, *Collections*, RCA Victor (1998)
Magical

Orff, *Carmina Burana*
Good for eliciting strong movement

Bach, Air on a G String, *The Great Dream Classics*, Great Classics Series, Delta Music PLC (1998)
Good for eliciting heavy movement

Mozart, Clarinet Concerto in A Major, *The Great Dream Classics* (1998)
Good for eliciting light movements

Balanesque Quartet, *Possessed*, Mute Records Ltd (1992)
Sharp,definite, industrial

Bert Kaempfert, *Roses*, tracks 10-14, Karusell
Playful

Bach, *Brandenburg Concerto No. 3- Allegro*
Dramatic, stormy, energetic

Various artists, *Tealands*, Putumayo World Music
Subdued classical

Sidney Berlin Ragtime Band, *Doop Doop*, Liberation Records (1994)
Energetic, fun and wacky music good for travelling and suddenness

Nature sounds

James Galway, *Songs of the Seashore*
Beautiful classical flute pieces with Japanese style and beach sounds

Tony O'Connor, *Sea Australia*, Studio Horizons Pty Ltd (1996)
Beach and wind sounds with ambient background rhythm

'Dugong Lullaby', 'Starfish Lagoon', Howlin Wind, *Dugong Lullaby*, Sony Masterworks (1995)
Atmospheric sea and forest themes

Steve Parrish, *Cry of the River Forest*, Steve Parrish Publishing (1996)
Australian nature and bird sounds

Children's music

Various artists, *Children's Party,* Musicband Ltd, Vol. 2 (2000)
Popular children's social dances

Various artists, *The Bird Dance and Other Party Favourites*, Mastertech (1998)
Popular children's social dances

Hi-5, *Jump & Jive with Hi-5,* Sony Wonder (2001)
pop-style Australian children's group

David Moses, *Okki Tokki Unga*, A&C Black Ltd. (1994)
Favourite children's songs to sing along

'There's a Wombat In My Room', Shenanigans, *There's A Wombat in My Room*,
Shenanigans, shenanigans@labryinth.net.au (1989)
Australian themed sing-along and social dance music

Relaxation/resting

Handel Water Music, *Great Classics Series,* Delta Music PLC
Flowing, watery

Pachelbel, *Canon and Gigue and other Baroque Masterpieces*, HNH International Ltd. (1989)

The Swoon Collections I, II and III, ABC Classics: Polygram (1998)
Good selection of classical favourites

Daniel Scott, *The Celtic Spirit*, Classic Fox Records (2000)
Also available with accompanying book of poems

K.C. Wang, *Chinese Bamboo Flute Songs*, Dex Audio (1996)
Lyrical Chinese style flute music

Enya, *Paint The Sky With Stars,* Warner Music UK (1997)
Hauntingly beautiful melodies accompanied by Irish-Gaelic singer Enya

Nomade, *Hussein El Masry*, Iris Musique Productions France (1997)
Evocative Middle-Eastern music

'Out of African Skies', *Out of Africa* soundtrack
Floaty dreamy feeling, good for relaxation

'Danny Boy', 'Annie's Song', *The Wind Beneath My Wings,* James Galway,
The Ultimate James Galway, RCA Victor (1999)
Easy-listening favourites

Bibliography

Bachman, J. and Sluyter, D. (1988) 'Reducing inappropriate behaviours of developmentally delayed adults using antecedent aerobic dance exercises', *Research in Developmental Disabilities*, 9, 73–83.

Bartenieff, I. and Lewis, D. (1980) *Body Movement: Coping with the Environment*, New York: Gordon and Breach.

Batshaw, M.L. (2002) *Children with Disabilities*, 5th ed, Brookes: Maryland.

Beange, H., Lennox, N. and Parmenter, T. (1999) 'Health targets for people with an intellectual disability', *Journal of Intellectual and Developmental Disability*, December, 283–97.

Beange, H., McElduff, A., and Baker, W. (1995) 'Medical disorders of adults with mental retardation: a population study', *American Journal on Mental Retardation*, 99, 595–604.

Benjamin, A. (2001), *Making An Entrance,* Routledge: London.

Berry, P., Groeneweg, G., Gibson, D. and Brown, R.I. (1984) 'Mental development of adults with Down syndrome', *American Journal of Mental Deficiency,* 89, 252–256.

Block, M. (2000) *A teacher's guide to including students with disabilities in general physical education* 2ed. Brookes: Maryland.

Blom, L. and Chaplin, L. (1988) *The Moment of Movement*, University of Pittsburg Press: Pittsburg.

Bond, K. (1994) 'How wild things tamed gender distinctions', *JOPERD*: February, 28–33.

Bond, K. (1999) *Class notes*, University of Melbourne.

Boswell, B. (1993) 'Effects of movement sequences and creative dance on balance of children with mental retardation', *Perceptual and Motor Skills*, 77, 3, 1290.

Boswell, B. (1993) 'Rhythmic movement and music for adolescents with severe and profound disabilities', *Music Therapy Perspectives*, 11, 1, 37–41.

Brown, M.B., Bayer, M.B. and Brown, P.M. (1992) *Empowerment and Developmental Handicaps: Choices and Quality of Life,* Captus Press: Toronto.

Brown, R. (1995) 'Social life, dating and marriage', in Nadel, L. and Rosenthal, D. (eds.) *Down Syndrome: Living and Learning in the Community*, (Proceedings of the Fifth International Down Syndrome Conference), Wiley-Liss: New York.

Bullen, P. and Onyx, J. (1998) *Measuring Social Capital in Five Communities in New South Wales: A Practitioner's Guide*, Management Alternatives.

Carnaby, S. (1999) *Designs for Living: A Comparative Approach to Normalization for the New Millennium,* Ashgate: USA.

Catalano R.F., Hawkins J. D. (1996) 'The social development model: A theory of anti-social behavior', in Hawkins, J.D., *Delinquency and Crime: Current Theories*, 9th edn, New York: Cambridge, 149–97.

Cathels, B.A., and Reddihough, D.S. (1993) 'The health care of young adults with cerebral palsy', *Medical Journal of Australia*, 15, 444–6.

Center, J., Beange, H., and McElduff, A. (1998) 'People with developmental disability have an increased prevalence of osteoporosis: A population study', *American Journal on Mental Retardation*, 103, 1928.

Champagne, M.P., Walker-Hirsch, L. (1993) *The Circles Concept of Intimacy and Relationships*, Stanfield: California.

Chance, Sally (2000) 'Restless Dance Company', in Buchanan, L. (ed.) *Positive/Negative: Writings on Integrated Dance*, Accessible Arts: NSW.

Chappell, C. (2000) 'Flying creatures from man to machine', in Buchanan, L. (ed.) *Positive/Negative: Writings on Integrated Dance,* Accessible Arts: NSW.

Clark, J. (1998) 'Older adult exercise techniques' in Cotton, R. (ed.) *Exercise for Older Adults: ACE's Guide for Fitness Professionals*, American Council on Exercise: San Diego.

Corkum, M., Ryan, P. and Cotter, T. (2001), VicHealth Letter, Victorian Health Promotion Foundation: Melbourne, p. 2.

Dalton, A.J. (1995) 'Alzheimer Disease: A health risk of growing older with Down syndrome', in Nadel, L. and Rosenthal, D. (eds) *Down Syndrome: Living and Learning in the Community*, Proceedings of the Fifth International Down Syndrome Conference, Wiley-Liss: New York.

Dean, O. (1993) 'The effective use of humour in human resource development', in J.W. Pfeiffer (ed.) *The 1993 Annual Developing Human Resources,* Pfeiffer and Company: San Diego.

Dell, C. (1977) *A Primer for Movement Description*, Dance Notation Bureau: New York.

Department of Human Services (1997), *Intellectual Disability: Some Questions and Answers,* Department of Human Services: Victoria.

Department of Human Services, (2002), State Disability Plan – The Key to Inclusion, at www.dhs.vic.gov.au/disability.

Driedger, D. (1989) *The Last Civil Rights Movement: Disabled Peoples' International*, New York: St. Martin's Press.

Dunphy, K. (1996) 'The transmission of culture through the arts' in Hillis, (ed.) *Conference Proceedings*, Greenmill World Dance: Melbourne.

Dunphy, K. (1999a) 'Dance and intellectual disability', in Guthrie, J. Loughlin, E. and Albiston, D (eds). *Dance Therapy Collections 2*, DTAA: Australia, 8–13.

Dunphy, K. (1999b) 'A creative arts program for incarcerated women', *International Journal of Psychotherapy in the Arts*, 26, 1, 35–43.

Dykens, E.M., Hodapp, R.M., Finucane, B.M. (2000) *Genetics and Mental Retardation Syndromes*, Brookes: Maryland.

Eckersley, R. (1999) *Quality of Life in Australia: An Analysis of Public Perceptions,* The Australia Institute: Canberra.

Exiner, J. and Kelynack, D. (1994) *Dance Therapy Re-defined: A Body Approach to*

Therapeutic Dance, Charles C. Thomas: Springfield.

Feder, B. and Feder, E. (1998) *The Art and Science of Evaluation in the Arts Therapies– How Do You Know What's Working?*, C.C. Thomas: Springfield.

Fiske, E. (ed) (1999) *Champions of Change—the impact of the arts on learning*, Arts Education Partnership: Washington, USA, at http://aep-arts.org/Champions.

Fitt, S. (1980) 'Simplified movement behaviour analysis as a basis for designing dance activities for the handicapped', in Fitt, S. and Riordan, A.(eds) *Focus on Dance IX: Dance for the handicapped*. AAPERD: Virginia.

Forssman, H. and Akesson, H. (1970) 'Mortality of the mentally deficient: A study of 12,903 institutionalized subjects', *Journal of Mental Deficiency Research*, 14, 276–94.

Freundlich, B.M., Pike, L., Schwartz, V. (1989), 'Dance and music for children with autism', *JOPERD*, Nov./Dec., 50–3.

Geeves, T. (1990) *Safe Dance Project Report*, Ausdance: Australia.

Geeves, T. (1997) *Safe Dance II*, Ausdance: Australia.

Guthrie, J. (2000) 'Movement assessment tools', *Dance Therapy Association of Australia Newsletter*, 7, 4, 4–5.

Guthrie, J. and Roydhouse, J. (1988) *Come and Join The Dance*, Hyland House: Melbourne.

Hartley (1995) *Wisdom of the Body Moving: An Introduction to Body Mind Centering*, North Atlantic Books: CA

Hawkes, J. (2001) *The Fourth Pillar of Sustainability: Culture's Essential Role in Public Planning*, Common Ground Publishing: Australia.

Hayden, M.F. (1998) 'Mortality among people with mental retardation living in the United States: Research review and policy application', *Mental Retardation*, 36, 345–359.

Hill, H. (2000), 'Notes from the Net', *Dance Therapy Association of Australia Newsletter*, 7, 3, 2–3.

Hill, H. (2001) *Invitation to the Dance*, University of Stirling: Scotland.

Hughes, Ginnet and Curphy, (1998), *Leadership: Enhancing the Lessons of Experience*, Richard D. Irwin Inc. Illinois.

Hugill, T. (1992), 'Theatre Unlimited and The Prime Movers', *Contact Quarterly*, 17, 1, 33–4.

Joy, R. (2000) *JustUs: Drama in the Community*, City of Port Phillip: Melbourne.

Joy, R. and Art of Difference Festival Steering Committee (eds) (2002) *Art of Difference Festival Report*, Gasworks: Melbourne.

Keating, C. (2002) *Evaluating Community Arts and Community Well Being*, Arts Victoria and VicHealth: Melbourne, at www.vichealth.vic.gov.au.

Kounin, J.S. (1941a) 'Experimental studies of rigidity: the measurement of rigidity in normal and feeble-minded persons', *Character and Personality*, 9, 251–72.

Kounin, J.S. (1941b) 'Experimental studies of rigidity: the explanatory power of the concept of rigidity as applied to feeble-mindedness', *Character and Personality*, 9, 273–82.

Kounin, J.S. (1948) 'The meaning of rigidity: A reply to Heinz Werner', *Psychological Review*, 55, 157–166.

Lasseter, J., Privette, G., Brown, C. and Duer, J. (1989) 'Dance as a treatment approach with a multi-disabled child: Implications for school counseling', *School Counselor*, vol. 36, 4, 310–15.

Leah, L. (2000) 'Developing a language for working in movement and dance', *DTAA Newsletter*, 7,1, 4–6.

Leventhal, M (1980) 'Dance therapy as treatment of choice for the emotionally disturbed and learning disabled child', *JOPER*, Sept., 33–5.

Leventhal, M. (1982) 'Movement and growth: Dance therapy for the special child', *American Journal of Dance Therapy*, 5, 74–5.

Levete, G. (1982) *No Handicap to Dance*, Horizon Books: UK.

Levy, F. (1988) *Dance Movement Therapy: A Healing Art*, AAHPERD: Virginia.

Lewin, K. (1935), *A Dynamic Theory of Personality*, McGraw-Hill, New York.

Lewis, C.B. and Campanelli, L.C. (1990), *Health Promotion and Exercise for Older Adults: An Instructor's Guide*, Aspen Publishers Inc: Maryland.

Lishman, J. (1985) 'Movement education and severely subnormal children: A review of the literature', *Early Childhood Development and Care*, 21, 1–3, 135–253.

Loman and Merman, (1996), 'Dance therapy as treatment of choice for the emotionally disturbed and learning disabled child', *Journal of Physical Health and Recreation*, Sept, 33–5.

Lovis, D. (1992), 'Prime Movers', *Contact Quarterly*, Winter, 33–4.

Lowenfeld, B. and Brittain, W.L. (1964) *Creative and Mental Growth*, Macmillan: NewYork.

Lowenfeld, B. and Brittain, W.L. (1964) *Creative and Mental Growth*, Macmillan: NewYork.

McCurrach, I. and Darnley, B. (1999) *Special Needs, Special Talents: Drama for People with Learning Disabilities*, Jessica Kingsley: UK.

Mead, J. (1999) *Dancing Communities: A Handbook of Community Dance*, Ausdance: Victoria.

Mettler, B. (1990) 'Creative dance: Art or therapy?', *American Journal of Dance Therapy*, 12, 2, 95–100.

Miller, S.G. (1984) *Music Therapy for Speech Impaired Children*, Project Music Monograph series, 2nd ed, p. 2.

Moore, C-L. and Yamamoto, K. (1988) *Beyond Words: Movement Observation and Analysis*, Gordon and Breach: New York.

Morrish (1999) Class notes, University of Melbourne.

Murrow, L. (1997) *Dance/movement therapy: Core values and assumptions*, course notes, RMIT, Melbourne.

Murrow, L. (1998), 'Conference 1997: Dance/movement therapy supervision', *Dance Therapy Association of Australia Newsletter,* 5, 3, 8–9.

Nachmanovitch, J. (1990) *Improvisation: Free Play in Life and Art,* J.P. Archer: Los Angeles.

Nirje, B. (1969) 'The normalization principle and its human management implications', in R. B. Kugel and W. Wolfensberger (eds), *Changing Residential Patterns for the Mentally Retarded,* Washington, DC: President's Committee on Mental Retardation, 227–254.

North, M. (1971) *Introduction to Movement Study and Teaching,* McDonalds-Evans: UK.

North, M. (1995) 'Catch the pattern', *American Journal of Dance Therapy,* 17, 1, 5–14.

O'Brien, K.E., Tate, K., Zaharia, E.S. (1991) 'Mortality in a large southeastern facility for persons with mental retardation', *American Journal of Mental Retardation,* 95, 397–403.

Ohwaki, S. (1976) 'An assessment of dance therapy to improve retarded adults' body image', *Perceptual and Motor Skills,* 43, 3, 1122.

Owen, A. (1999), 'Using Laban Movement Analysis to assess progress in dance therapy', in Guthrie, J., Loughlin, E., and Albiston, D. (eds) *Dance Therapy Collections 2,* DTAA: Australia, 31-36.

Rimmer, J.H., Braddock, D. and Fujijura, G. (1993) 'Prevalence of obesity in adults with mental retardation: Implications for health promotion and disease prevention', *Mental Retardation,* 31, 105–10.

Rimmer, J. (1998) 'Common health challenges faced by older adults', in Cotton, R. (ed,) *Exercise for Older Adults,* American Council on Exercise: San Diego.

Riordan, A. (1989), 'Sunrise Wheels', *JOPERD,* Nov–Dec 89, 62–4.

Roizen, N., Luke, A., Sutton, M., and Schoeller, D.A. (1995) 'Obesity and nutrition in children with Down Syndrome', in Nadel, L. and Rosenthal, D. (eds) *Down Syndrome: Living and Learning in the Community,* Proceedings of the Fifth International Down Syndrome Conference, Wiley-Liss: New York.

Rowitz, L.and Jurkowski, E. (1995) 'The myths and realities of depression and Down Syndrome' in Nadel, L. and Rosenthal, D. (eds.) *Down Syndrome: Living and Learning in the Community,* Proceedings of the Fifth International Down Syndrome Conference, Wiley-Liss: New York.

Schlusser, A. (2000) Perceptions of improvisational performance from a group of artists with intellectual disabilities, unpublished MA thesis, University of Melbourne: Australia

Schmais, C. (1974) 'Dance therapy in perspective', in Mason. K. (ed.) *Focus on Dance VII: Dance Therapy,* AAPERD: Virginia.

Selikowitch, M. (1992) 'Down Syndrome: The facts', in Brown, R.I. (ed.) *The 1992 National Conference of the Canadian Down Syndrome Society,* Canadian Down Syndrome Society and Rehabilitation Studies: University of Calgary, 3–25.

Sharkey, B. (1990) *The Physiology of Fitness,* Human Kinetics Publishers: Illinois.

Shepperdson, B. (1995) 'Two longitudinal studies of the abilities of people with Down's syndrome', *Journal of Intellectual Disability Research,* 39, 419–31.

Silk, G. (1989) 'Creative movement for people who are developmentally disabled', *JOPERD*, Nov–Dec. 89, 56–58.

Stabler, J., Stabler, J. and Karger, R. (1977) Evaluation of paintings of non-retarded and retarded persons by judges with and without art training in American Journal of Mental Deficiency, 81, 502-503

Stamatelos, T. and Mott. D. (1983a) *Writing as Therapy: Motivational Activities for the Developmentally Delayed*, Columbia University Teachers' College Press: New York.

Stamatelos, T., and Mott, D. (1985) 'Creative potential among persons labelled developmentally delayed', *The Arts in Psychotherapy*, 12, 2, 101–13.

St George, F. (1994) *The Stretching Handbook: 10 Steps to Muscle Fitness,* Simon and Schuster: Australia.

Stinson, S. (1988) *Dance for Young Children: Finding the Magic in Movement*, AAPERD: Virginia.

Stinson, S. (1990) 'Dance and the developing child', in W. Stinson, (ed.) *Moving and Learning in the Young Child*, AAHPERD: Virginia.

Strauss, D. and Eyman, R. (1996) 'Mortality of people with mental retardation in California with and without Down syndrome, 1986–1991', *American Journal on Mental Retardation,* 100, 643–53.

Thompson, S. and Hoekenga, S.J. (1998) 'Understanding and motivating older adults', in Cotton, R. (ed.) (1998), *Exercise for Older Adults,* American Council on Exercise: San Diego.

Threlfall, C. (2002) '*News From Afar*' seminar, Arts Access: Melbourne, 30 April.

Tipple (1975) 'Dance therapy and education program', *Journal of Leisurability,* 2, 4, 9–12.

US Surgeon-General's Report, (1996), *Physical Activity and Health*, US Government Printing Office: Washington DC.

Wehmeyer, M. and Schwartz, M. (1998) 'The relationship between self-determination and quality of life for adults with mental retardation', *Education and Training in Mental Retardation and Developmental Disabilities,* 33, 1, 3–12.

West, R. (1996) 'Kew fire shows the tragedy of those shut away', *The Age*, 20 April, p. 19.

Williams, D. (2001) *Defining the Domain: Valuing Arts and Culture*, in culture@com.unity conference proceedings, UTS: Sydney.

Wishart, L. (2000) *Class notes,* University of Melbourne.

Wolfensberger, W. (ed.) (1972) *Normalization: The Principle of Normalization*, National Institute on Mental Retardation: Toronto.

World Health Organization, (1997), 'The Heidelberg Guidelines for promoting physical activity among older persons', *Journal of Aging and Physical Activity*, 5, 1, 2–8.

Worth, K. (2000) 'Integrated dance workshop stories', in Buchanan, L. (ed) *Positive/Negative: Writings on Integrated Dance*, Accessible Arts: NSW.

Yang, Q., Rasmussen, SA., Friedman, JM. (2002) *Mortality associated with Down's Syndrome in the USA from 1983-1997: a population based study*, Lancet 23:359, 9311: 1019-25.

Zagelbaum, V. and Rubino, M. (1991) 'Combined dance/movement, art, and music therapies with a developmentally delayed psychiatric client in a day treatment setting', *The Arts in Psychotherapy,* 18, pp. 139–48.

Further reading

Bornell, D.G. (1988) 'Movement is individuality: An inter-abilities approach using dance taps', *Music Therapy*, 4, 1, 98–105.

Brown, R.I. and Timmons, V. (1993) *Quality of Life: Adults and Adolescents with Disabilities*, Exceptionality Education: Canada.

Bunney, J. (1977) 'Dance therapy', in Valletutti, P. and Christoplos, F. (eds) *Interdisciplinary Approaches to Human Services*, University Park Press: Maryland.

Capute, A.J. (1996) *Developmental Disabilities in Infancy and Childhood*, 2nd ed, Brookes: Maryland.

Cotton, R. (ed.) (1998) *Exercise for Older Adults: ACE's Guide for Fitness Professionals*, American Council on Exercise: San Diego.

Firth, H. and Rapley, M. (1990) *From Acquaintance to Friendship: Issues for People with Learning Disabilities,* Kidderminster: BIMH Publications.

Hill, H. (2001) *Invitation to the Dance,* University of Stirling: Scotland.

Jancar, J., and Speller, C.J. (1994) 'Fatal intestinal obstruction in the mentally handicapped', *Journal of Intellectual Disability Research*, 38, 413–22.

Kapit, W. and Elson, L.M. (1977) *The Anatomy Coloring Book*, Harper and Row: New York.

Kestenberg, J. (1967) *The Role of Movement Patterns in Development*, Dance Notation Bureau: New York.

Koegel, R.L. and Koegel, L.K. (1995) *Teaching Children with Autism: Strategies for Initiating Positive Interaction and Improving Learning Opportunities*, Brookes: Maryland.

Levinson, B. (director) (1998) *Rainman* (motion picture), Guber-Peters/United Artists, Los Angeles.

Lewis, P. and Loman, S. (1990) *The Kestenberg Movement Profile: Its Past, Present and Future Applications and Future Directions,* Keene Antioch NH: New England Graduate School.

Loman, S. and Merman, H. (1996) 'The KMP: A tool for dance/movement therapy', *American Journal of Dance Therapy*, 18, 1, 29–49.

Nadel, L. and Rosenthal, D. (eds.) (1995) *Down Syndrome: Living and Learning in the Community,* Proceedings of the Fifth International Down Syndrome Conference, Wiley-Liss: New York.

Newton, R. (1992), *Down's Syndrome*, Optima Books: UK.

Payne, H. (1994) *Creative Movement and Dance in Group Work*, Winslow Press: UK.

Pueschel, S.M. (1997) *Adolescents with Down Syndrome*, Brookes: Maryland.

Pueschel, S.M. (2001) *A Parent's Guide to Down Syndrome*, Brookes: Maryland.

Quill, K.A. (2000) *Do-Watch-Listen-Say, Social and Communication Intervention for Children with Autism,* Brookes: Maryland.

Smith, S. (1987) *Extending Self-Concept and Social Behaviour Skills Though the Circle Concept,* Social Biology Resource Centre: Melbourne.

St. George, F. (1992) *The Muscle Fitness Book,* Simon and Schuster: Australia.

Strauss, D. Eyman, R.K., and Grossman, H.J. (1996) 'Predictors of mortality in children with severe mental retardation: the effect of placement', *American Journal of Public Health,* 86, 1429–32.

Warburg, M., and Rattleff, J. (1992) 'Treatable visual impairment. A study of 778 consecutive patients with mental handicap placed in sheltered workshops', in J.J. Roosendahl (ed.) *Mental Retardation and Medical Care,* Uitgeverij Kerkebosch, Zeist, 350–6.

Williams, D. (1996) *Creating Social Capital,* Community Arts Network of South Australia: Adelaide.

Index

Notes

Notes

Notes

Notes

Notes

Notes

Notes

Notes

Notes

Notes